The Long Covid
self-help guide

The Long Covid

self-help guide

Practical ways to manage symptoms

From the Specialists at the
Post-Covid Clinic, Oxford

GREEN TREE
LONDON · OXFORD · NEW YORK · NEW DELHI · SYDNEY

GREEN TREE
Bloomsbury Publishing Plc
50 Bedford Square, London, WC1B 3DP, UK
29 Earlsfort Terrace, Dublin 2, Ireland

BLOOMSBURY, GREEN TREE and the Green Tree logo
are trademarks of Bloomsbury Publishing Plc

First published in Great Britain 2022

For legal purposes the Acknowledgements on p. 196 constitute an extension
of this copyright page. Image on p. 187 © Getty Images.

A catalogue record for this book is available from the British Library

Library of Congress Cataloguing-in-Publication data has been applied for

ISBN: TPB: 978-1-3994-0202-6; eBook: 978-1-3994-0201-9; ePdf: 978-1-3994-0200-2

2 4 6 8 10 9 7 5 3 1

Typeset in Minion Pro by seagulls.net
Printed and bound in Great Britain by CPI Group (UK) Ltd, Croydon CR0 4YY

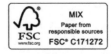

To find out more about our authors and books visit
www.bloomsbury.com and sign up for our newsletters

CONTENTS

THE CONTRIBUTORS

Dr Emily Fraser, Consultant in Respiratory Medicine, Oxford University NHS Foundation Trust; Clinical Lead for the Post-Covid Assessment Clinic, Oxford.

Dr Anton Pick, Consultant in Rehabilitation Medicine; Clinical Lead at the Oxford Centre for Enablement; Clinical Lead for Long Covid, NHS England: South East of England.

Rachael Rogers, Specialist Occupational Therapist; Clinical Lead of the Community Chronic Fatigue Service, Oxfordshire; member of the Post-Covid Assessment Clinic and rehabilitation team, Oxford.

Emma Tucker, Specialist Respiratory Physiotherapist and Clinical Lead for the Post-Covid Rehabilitation Service in Oxford Health NHS Foundation Trust.

Dr Daniel Zahl, Consultant Clinical Psychologist; CBT therapist and supervisor; member of the Post-Covid Assessment Clinic, Oxford.

Dr Suleman Latif, Specialist Registrar in Sport and Exercise Medicine, Oxford.

Ruth Tyerman, Specialist Vocational Rehabilitation Occupational Therapist; member of the Post-Covid Assessment Clinic, Oxford.

Dr Christopher Turnbull, NIHR Clinical Lecturer in Respiratory Medicine, University of Oxford and the Oxford University Hospitals NHS Foundation Trust.

Christine Kelly, Founder of charity AbScent; Research Associate at the University of Reading; Research Fellow at the Centre for the Study of the Senses, Institute of Philosophy, University of London.

Dr Helen Davies, Consultant Respiratory Physician; Clinical Lead for the Pleural and Post-Covid Respiratory Services, University Hospital of Wales.

Emily Jay, Clinical Specialist Physiotherapist with an Interest in Vestibular Rehabilitation, South London and the Maudsley NHS Trust.

Lisa Burrows, Consultant Physiotherapist and clinical lead of the ENT Balance Clinic, Mersey Care NHS Foundation Trust.

Dr Andrew Lewis, Clinical Lecturer in Cardiovascular Medicine, University of Oxford.

Dr Rohan Wijesurendra, Clinical Lecturer in Cardiovascular Medicine, University of Oxford; Cardiology Registrar at the Oxford University Hospitals NHS Foundation Trust.

Dr Julia Newton, Consultant in Rheumatology/Sport and Exercise Medicine (SEM), Oxford University Hospitals Trust; Senior Sports Physician, English Institute of Sport.

Dr Christopher Speers, Consultant in Sport and Exercise Medicine, Nuffield Orthopaedic Centre, Oxford.

Dr Andy Tyerman, Consultant Clinical Neuropsychologist, Trustee of Headway UK and the Vocational Rehabilitation Association.

With additional contributions from:
Dr Kim Rajappan, Consultant Cardiologist, Oxford University NHS Foundation Trust; Dr Annabel Nickol, Consultant in Sleep Medicine, Oxford University NHS Foundation Trust; Dr Tylan Yukselen, Consultant in Psychological Medicine, Oxford University NHS Foundation Trust; Dr Nick Talbot, Respiratory Consultant, Oxford University NHS Foundation Trust; Professor Jane Parker, Founder and Director of the Flavour Centre, University of Reading; The Oxfordshire Post-Covid Rehabilitation team: Victoria Masey, Kerrie Crowley, Catherine Clayton, Rebecca Prower, Rachel Lardner, Amanda Neophytou, Lisa Johnson, Jill Brooks, Kelly Mclaughlin; Lizzie Grillo on behalf of Physiotherapy for Breathing Pattern Disorders; Tania Clifton-Smith on behalf of Bradcliff Breathing™ methods.

Introduction

You are probably reading this book because you or someone you love is suffering from Long Covid. We do not have all the answers yet, but we have written this to share with you our experiences and knowledge so that you may start feeling better. This book is the product of a collaborative effort by a group of healthcare professionals, many of whom have been supporting people suffering from Long Covid since it first emerged during 2020. Working alongside our patients, we have identified ways to help people manage the symptoms of Long Covid. We hope this book will provide you with effective, easy-to-understand and practical guidance. The recommendations are tried and tested and, through our work in the Post-Covid Assessment Clinic, Oxford (also known as the Oxford Long Covid clinic), have already helped many hundreds of patients.

How to use the book

Our goal is to equip you with insights and tools to empower you to move forward, manage setbacks, and make progress towards your recovery. The book is divided into chapters, each covering common problems encountered by the people we have met in the Long Covid clinic. You can read the chapters in order or you may find it useful to dip in and out, identifying sections covering the particular challenges you are struggling with at the moment. You may want to use the book to help explain your experience to your loved ones and friends or perhaps even to your employer or colleagues. We encourage you to highlight relevant passages, annotate the book with your own thoughts and lessons, or perhaps listen to the audiobook as you go about your day-to-day life. Your symptoms may limit how much you can absorb in one sitting. That is OK. Take your time. Use this book to navigate your own path to recovery.

Look out for stories from patients throughout the book – they have had a very similar experience to you, so you'll find their tips and suggestions very helpful as you manage your own recovery.

The emergence of the Covid-19 pandemic and Long Covid

The pandemic seemed to emerge out of nowhere. Towards the end of 2019 we started hearing unfamiliar terms in the news, such as 'lockdown' and 'contact tracing'. These buzzwords have now become ubiquitous. When the first stories emerged out of China, they seemed distant and abstract for many of us. However, very quickly, the virus landed on our shores and our reality changed. Populations all over the world faced lockdowns and 'stay at home' orders. All of a sudden, activities that defined everyday life, such as sharing time with friends and family, playing sports together, even going shopping, all carried risk. Our way of life changed overnight in ways that this generation had never known or expected. Everything familiar seemed uncertain and scary. Death and suffering, both of which we often try to ignore, were suddenly pervasive – in daily announced statistics, newsreels, online images and stories on social media. Images of hospitals overflowing, of exhausted healthcare professionals, of overfilled mortuaries were inescapable.

As we stayed home to avoid contracting or spreading the disease, many of us unable to turn away from the ceaseless onslaught of alarming news, a parallel story began emerging. A story of persistent and varied symptoms that long outlasted the initial infection. Was this Covid-19 pandemic more than an acute viral illness? What was this new, tenacious condition that some people were experiencing? Its name was coined by a sufferer before healthcare professionals even recognised its existence – Long Covid. Many of the people suffering from it called themselves 'long-haulers'.

Long Covid: From personal experience to social media

This global pandemic has indeed brought us more than just a dangerous acute viral disease. The first public rumblings of this other condition were on social media. People started sharing their experiences of persisting, unexplained symptoms, including overwhelming fatigue, breathlessness, palpitations, muscle pains, brain fog and dizziness. Sufferers described their struggles to find healthcare professionals who would take their experiences seriously. Many people told troubling stories of feeling disbelieved or even 'gaslit' by healthcare professionals. Unable to find the help they needed, they found solidarity and support in social media groups. After what seemed like far too long, media outlets and policymakers eventually started to pay attention, and sufferers finally started to feel heard. In some places, specialist clinics and services were set up to offer support and treatment. The Oxford Long Covid clinic was one of the earliest of these services in the UK.

How does medical science respond to a new disease?

It takes an average of seven years for scientific discoveries to translate into approved medical treatments. To develop a vaccine and navigate through the various phases of clinical trials and regulatory approvals normally takes around 10 to 15 years. Compared to the normal pace of progress, this pandemic has been an extreme outlier. The first breakthrough was the identification of the virus itself. This took scientists in China only one week. The new virus was named SARS-CoV-2, and the disease it caused was called Covid-19. Overnight, those names were everywhere. This was a vital first step but shed little light on how to contain the virus or how to treat people suffering from the disease it was causing. As the pandemic spread, the focus of the entire global scientific community soon converged on deciphering this new common enemy. Public health measures, such as social distancing, 'stay at home' orders, masking, quarantining and contact tracing, were instituted in many places to control the spread of the virus. Very soon, healthcare professionals were trialling possible treatments for people afflicted with the virus. Treatments fell in and out of favour as evidence was gathered at breakneck speed. Never before, on such a grand scale and with such urgent importance, had we witnessed science unfolding in real time like this. Vaccines for Covid-19 were developed, tested and approved in less than a year. Incredible progress on managing this pandemic has been made already and scientists are increasingly redirecting their attention to understanding Long Covid.

The medical science of Long Covid

While many theories about Long Covid have been proposed, the science underlying it remains murky. Long Covid appears to be quite arbitrary in who it afflicts. People who were extremely unwell during their acute Covid-19 illness, including some who were hospitalised and underwent invasive and sometimes life-saving treatments such as mechanical ventilation, are affected, as are people who suffered only mild acute symptoms. Medical testing sometimes diagnoses conditions such as hypothyroidism or vitamin D deficiency that might at least partially explain some symptoms. For many sufferers, however, the results of standard medical investigations do not fully account for the large array of their symptoms. So, what exactly causes Long Covid? Why do some people develop it and others not? Why are the symptoms different in different people? How can we predict how long symptoms will last? Medical scientists are busy at work trying to answer these questions. Theories have been proposed and are being tested. Treatments have been suggested and are being trialled. At the time of writing, no medications have been licensed for use in this condition. However, fortunately, drug treatments are not the only way we manage medical conditions.

What is 'whole person' care?

Medical science has made incredible progress in understanding, diagnosing and treating diseases, but there is still much that we do not understand. This fact is quite difficult to accept for healthcare professionals and patients alike. Doctors are not always effective at navigating uncertainty with their patients. Some Long Covid sufferers have reported feeling their experience has not been validated by their doctor. Some have even left consultations feeling like they have not been believed. Regardless of whether or not we are able to explain their cause, your symptoms and your suffering are absolutely real. Despite all that we have yet to understand, there is much we can offer to help you.

Diseases are often described simplistically, as a broken or malfunctioning body. Healthcare, it might be suggested, is therefore simply aimed at finding the broken body parts and fixing them, much like a car mechanic does with a malfunctioning car. This formulation works perfectly for some conditions, such as broken bones, that are quite fixable. For many other conditions, however, for which there is no simple fix or cure, and Long Covid is only one among many of these, this perspective can be limiting and unhelpful. It does not take into consideration the individual, their environment and other factors that shape the unique suffering a disease might cause. A 'whole person' care approach considers the individual with the condition and the particular factors in their life that play a role in shaping their unique experience. It is this approach that opens the door to relieving suffering, when a quick fix is not readily available. We are all complex beings and our biology is shaped by our environment and the world in which we live, so we need to take that into account when managing complex conditions. The Oxford Long Covid clinic and many other Long Covid services recommend taking a 'whole person' approach to your treatment. Some of the recommendations and exercises in this book are aimed at directly relieving a specific symptom you might be experiencing, and others are aimed at focusing your attention, for a time, on more general ways to ease your suffering and improve your overall quality of life. We have found that approaching this condition from both angles works best to achieve the best possible outcomes.

SUMMARY

- The symptoms that you are experiencing with Long Covid are most likely impacting you in physical, emotional and social ways.

- Feeling unwell can impact on how we perceive ourselves, what we can and cannot do, how we behave and how we relate to those around us.

- This book is aimed at helping you with your own unique set of challenges, to start to find a way to feel better. Its purpose is to help signpost you to strategies and techniques for reducing the impact that Long Covid is having on your life.

- You are on an uncertain journey, but we hope that you find this book a worthy companion and guide as you travel towards recovery.

CHAPTER 1

What is Long Covid?

The term 'Long Covid' was created by people burdened with its symptoms. In this chapter, we look at how Long Covid is defined and describe some of the more common symptoms experienced.

'When I got Long Covid in March 2020, I was 38 and healthy. If you are anything like I was then, it is hard to understand how bad Long Covid is. I think we all have an instinct to look away, but please, it is important that you look.'

A recognised complication of Covid-19

The term 'Long Covid' is widely used to describe the presence of symptoms lasting for longer than four weeks after an episode of Covid-19. This is estimated to affect around 10 per cent of people, with symptoms that vary in extent and severity. Considering that recovery times for infections such as flu and pneumonia can span several months, it is not really surprising that many people do not feel 100 per cent four weeks after Covid. By 12 weeks, however, most people do feel better, although there remain a proportion (probably yourself included) who continue to be afflicted with symptoms that limit ordinary and everyday activities. It's difficult to gauge the exact percentage of people who suffer long term with symptoms from Covid because of the different ways that data is collected, but it is clear that the burden of Long Covid is immense, with hundreds of thousands of individuals affected in the UK alone.*

---

* Office of National Statistics Prevalence of ongoing symptoms following coronavirus (Covid-19) infection in the UK. https://www.ons.gov.uk/peoplepopulationandcommunity/ healthandsocialcare/healthandlifeexpectancies/datasets/prevalenceoflongcovidsymptoms andcovid19complications

Symptoms of Long Covid are diverse. Fatigue is the most frequently reported; other common symptoms include breathlessness, cognitive problems (including memory impairment and poor concentration), chest and body pains, dizziness, palpitations and persistent smell impairment, but there are many others. Interestingly, the severity of the initial infection does not seem to predict whether or not you will go on to develop Long Covid. Indeed, many people with Long Covid had a relatively mild infection.

Long Covid is now a recognised complication of Covid-19. However, its emergence took many healthcare professionals by surprise. The focus early on in the pandemic was on how best to prevent the spread of the virus, treat the acute infection and save as many lives as possible. Only months into the pandemic (many frustrated at how many months afterwards) did the huge public health implications of Long Covid became apparent.

In retrospect, Long Covid was fairly predictable for two reasons:

1. Viruses are recognised triggers for chronic post-viral fatigue syndromes (almost two-thirds of patients report an infective illness prior to developing myalgic encephalomyelitis (ME)/chronic fatigue syndrome (CFS)).
2. Other viral pandemics, such as influenza (highlighted as far back as the Spanish flu in 1918) and SARS (in 2003, caused by a similar coronavirus – SARS-CoV), are known to have resulted in long-term health problems similar to Long Covid, including fatigue, body pains and cognitive issues.

Defining Long Covid

The diagnosis of Long Covid is made on the basis of 'typical' symptoms after other possible causes have been excluded. No two cases of Long Covid are identical. While some people report one or two dominant symptoms, others experience multiple problems at the same time. Symptoms can be mild or severe and often wax and wane over time, with new ones emerging as others fade away. Some symptoms seem to cluster together, while others appear independently and out of the blue. The National Institute for Health Research (NIHR) has recorded over 205 symptoms, although there may be even more than this.

*'My symptoms are interlinked. Clearly, my worst cluster is
neuropsychiatric, including co-occurring headache, dizziness,
insomnia and anxiety, alongside brain fog.'*

The term 'Long Covid' was coined by the patients themselves before
the condition was fully recognised by the medical profession. It is still
the term most widely used and understood by both the public and the
medical community and has been adopted throughout this book. There
are, however, more formal definitions now in use. In the United Kingdom,
people who have symptoms after 12 weeks are referred to as having 'Post-
Covid-19 Syndrome'. This has been defined by the National Institute of
Clinical Excellence (NICE) and is described as:

'Ongoing symptoms after 12 weeks not explained by an alternative diagnosis. It usually presents with clusters of symptoms,
often overlapping, which can fluctuate and can affect any system
in the body.'*

More recently, after expert consensus (including large patient advocate
groups), the World Health Organization (WHO) has now officially named
Long Covid 'Post Covid-19 Condition' (PCC). This definition expands on
the one above; it includes the major symptoms, and recognises the impact
it has on daily life (but is otherwise very similar):

'Post-Covid-19 condition occurs in individuals with a history of
probable or confirmed SARS-CoV2 infection, usually 3 months
from the onset of Covid-19 with symptoms that last at least
2 months and cannot be explained by an alternative diagnosis.

'Common symptoms include fatigue, shortness of breath,
cognitive dysfunction but also others which generally have an
impact of everyday functioning. Symptoms may be new onset,
following initial recovery from an acute Covid-19 episode, or

---

* NICE (2021) 'Covid-19 rapid guideline: managing the long-term effects of Covid-19'.
https://www.nice.org.uk/guidance/ng188/resources/covid19-rapid-guideline-managing-
the-longterm- effects-of-covid19-pdf-51035515742

persist from the initial illness. Symptoms may also fluctuate or relapse over time. A separate definition may be applicable for children.'*

Other terms include Post-Acute Covid-19 Syndrome (PACS) and the less catchy Post-Acute Sequelae of Covid-19 (PASC). They all refer to the same condition.

What causes symptoms in Long Covid?

The truth is that we don't yet know the answer.

However, we do recognise that Long Covid is not due to a single problem or 'abnormality' and the reasons people continue to experience symptoms months after developing Covid-19 differ. Some of these are more straightforward to understand than others, particularly if you were severely unwell during the infection and required admission to hospital.

Long Covid after hospitalisation

We recognise that longer-term symptoms are not uncommon after severe illness. For example, prolonged stays in Intensive Care are associated with generalised loss of muscle and often lead to persisting weakness. Cognitive problems occur after severe illness due to the huge impact of the illness itself as well as the life-saving treatment you will have received. Undertaking physical activity may also be more difficult due to breathing problems caused by lung damage following severe Covid pneumonia. Unsurprisingly, after life-threatening illness, people are at higher risk of psychological problems such as anxiety and post-traumatic stress disorder due to harrowing experiences they have been through.

Admission to hospital with Covid-19 is usually associated with more severe infection. In these cases, lingering symptoms are therefore not unexpected. A large study from Wuhan in China reported that most people discharged from hospital had at least one ongoing symptom at six

---

* World Health Organization (2021) 'A clinical case definition of post Covid-19 condition by a Delphi consensus'. https://www.who.int/publications/i/item/WHO-2019-nCoV-Post_ COVID-19_ condition-Clinical_case_definition-2021.

Symptom	Percentage of people affected at 6 months
Fatigue	63
Breathlessness on exercise*	26
Sleep difficulties	26
Hair loss	22
Smell disturbance	11
Palpitations	9
Joint pain	9
Decreased appetite	8
Taste disturbance	7
Dizziness	6
Diarrhoea or vomiting	5
Chest pain	5
Sore throat or difficulty swallowing	4

TABLE 1: A list of the most common symptoms reported by 1733 individuals six months after being discharged from hospital following treatment for Covid-19. (Huang et al., *The Lancet* 397(10270), January 2021, pp. 220–232).

* Findings based on a breathlessness score called the modified Medical Research Council (mMRC) dyspnoea scale.

months. The most common symptoms were fatigue, muscle weakness and sleep disturbance (table 1 gives the full list of symptoms).

While the severity of infection can offer some explanation for persisting symptoms, it certainly does not explain the full picture. The Wuhan study, for example, showed that even people with milder Covid-19 who were admitted to hospital (but did not receive oxygen therapy or go to critical care) reported persisting symptoms at a frequency not dissimilar to those who were severely ill.

Long Covid after milder infection

Long Covid after milder infection is still poorly understood. Researchers have flagged 'risk factors' that suggest some groups of people are more susceptible to longer-term consequences, but they don't explain why some people of the same gender, background and health status make a complete recovery while others struggle with symptoms for months after becoming unwell.

It is also not clear why symptoms can evolve and change over time. We often see people in clinic who describe getting better, even returning to work and exercise, only to relapse with Long Covid symptoms weeks or months later. This is a common enough phenomenon to be recognised within the World Health Organization definition of the condition (*see* page 9). Furthermore, echoing our experience, a UK survey found that three-quarters of people with Long Covid develop symptoms over time that were not present or noticeable during their initial illness.

> 'Long Covid feels like a hex. Your body and brain are wrong, in different ways on different days, unpredictable and unsettling. On the good days you doubt yourself; on the bad, you doubt everything. The illness is capricious, boundless and wicked.'

So it's clear that the explanation for persisting symptoms in people who had a milder illness is less straightforward, raising more questions than answers at the moment for people with Long Covid and medical professionals alike.

Despite the uncertainty surrounding this condition, there are several proposed theories of Long Covid currently being researched. These include (but are certainly not limited to):

- **The triggering of an autoimmune disease process.** An autoimmune disease occurs when the immune system behaves abnormally and recognises certain cells and tissues in the body as 'foreign' and attacks them. Examples include rheumatoid arthritis and systemic lupus erythematosus ('lupus').
- **Persistent low-level inflammation.** Inflammation that continues weeks to months after becoming infected by Covid-19. One hypothesis is that low-level inflammation may be driven by the persistence of the virus or viral material at a concentration not detected by conventional tests.
- **Covid-induced neurological damage**. Some people affected by Long

Covid report symptoms that suggest parts of the nervous system might be malfunctioning. An inappropriately fast heart rate after minimal exertion, for example, suggests an impairment of the 'autonomic' nervous system, the part of the nervous system responsible for controlling automatic functions. How the virus causes these problems is not yet known, but this is a recogrnised phenomenon following other viral infections.

- **Multi-organ damage.** Studies using whole body magnetic resonance imaging (MRI) have found that in some people who have had Covid, abnormalities persist in different organs for months after the initial infection. The explanation for this is unknown, but one possibility is that damage is caused by inflammation or the presence of tiny clots ('microclots') within the smaller blood vessels supplying the affected organs. What has not been established, however, is a clear link between these MRI findings and the presence of symptoms.

Common symptoms of Long Covid

Over 200 symptoms have been reported by people suffering with Long Covid. There are several symptoms that are more frequently reported by sufferers. In our experience, fatigue, brain fog and breathlessness feature most prominently in the people we see in our clinic.

Pins and needles Headache

Hair and nail changes

Fatigue Loss of smell

Chest and body pains **Dizziness**

Tinnitis Cough **Breathlessness**

Palpitations Fever

Brain fog Anxiety

Sore throat

Sleep disturbance **Low mood**

Skin rashes

Gastrointestinal disturbance

Let's now look at the most common Long Covid symptoms. Practical advice and guidance about how to manage these symptoms is the subject of the rest of this book, broken down into key symptom chapters. The symptom list that follows is not exhaustive in any way but hopefully gives an insight into some of the more common problems we see in the Long Covid clinic and that may be affecting you.

Fatigue

'Fatigue is a useless description of the existential exhaustion I felt every day for at least a year. A flat battery that sleep barely touched. Like the most severe jet lag and hangover I've ever had, together. Every single day and night.'

Fatigue can be a crippling symptom and is experienced by most people with Long Covid (up to 80 per cent, in some surveys). Definitions of fatigue are varied but in Long Covid, people often describe a profound loss of energy and the feeling of extreme physical and mental tiredness or exhaustion. While fatigue is a normal sensation after exercise or a hard day's work, in Long Covid it can be unrelenting and made worse by tasks that would have previously seemed trivial. Many people suffering with Long Covid find that their fatigue and other symptoms worsen significantly after physical activity or exercise. This is known as post-exertional malaise (PEM).

There are many causes of fatigue and people may feel fatigued for more than one reason. Chronic disease, poor sleep quality, reduced physical exertion, anaemia and depression are some of the common causes of fatigue. Table 2 provides a list of some other common causes.

Fatigue can have a devastating impact on all aspects of your life. It can limit your ability to carry out your job, prevent you from being able to enjoy leisure activities, or even impair your ability to carry out the basic tasks of everyday living, such as washing and dressing. This can impact on your life in other ways, such as on your relationships, family life and financial situation. Those most severely affected may struggle to look after themselves or their children or other dependents. Fatigue can impact on your mood and well-being, with many people, unsurprisingly, developing low mood, depression or anxiety. Practical advice on managing fatigue and

Post-viral syndromes (including Long Covid, glandular fever)
Poor sleep
Medications (particularly some older antihistamines, beta blockers, antidepressants and painkillers e.g. morphine)
Substance use (including caffeine, alcohol, marijuana)
Anxiety, depression and PTSD
Rheumatological conditions, including fibromyalgia, systemic lupus erythematosus, rheumatoid arthritis
Endocrine disease (particularly hypothyroidism)
Anaemia
Chronic disease, including that affecting the heart, lungs, liver, kidneys and nervous system

TABLE 2: Common causes of fatigue that may be considered when clinically assessing people of Long Covid.

helping conserve energy is provided in chapter 2. Managing a return to exercise can be particularly difficult for those who suffer from post-exertional malaise. Guidance to help navigate this is offered in chapter 3.

> 'My own low points: early on, I collapsed, shaking, and was taken to A&E in an ambulance. A year later, I did not have the energy to leave the house. Formerly I was a marathon runner, but I brought on a bad relapse with a 700m walk.'

Memory and cognitive problems ('brain fog')

Cognitive problems are quite common following any severe illness. People admitted to intensive care are particularly susceptible. In fact, 'post-intensive care syndrome' (PICS) has been coined to describe the health problems people can struggle with after leaving intensive care, and this includes issues with memory, attention, problem-solving and complex tasks.

However, many people suffering from Long Covid had a relatively mild infection. So there is likely to be a different explanation for the cognitive problems, and this is an area of active investigation. Often called 'brain fog', symptoms relate to issues with memory, attention span, and processing of information. People we see in the clinic talk about a slowness of thought, forgetfulness and not being able to find the right word. Brain fog and fatigue often come hand in hand, with few people reporting one symptom without the other. There are practical strategies to help manage brain fog in chapters 2 and 8.

> 'Brain fog is a bit like being "extremely" sleep deprived –
> remember, sleep deprivation is literally a technique of torture – but
> you can't sleep off brain fog. It feels like being lost in a fog and
> sensing dark shapes...'

Breathlessness

The medical term for breathlessness (or shortness of breath) is dyspnoea. This is defined as 'difficult or laboured breathing', although people describe the sensation of breathlessness in many ways. Commonly used descriptions include:

- the feeling of chest tightness or pressure;
- having to work harder to take a breath;
- difficulty breathing in or a struggle to take a deep breath in;
- a conscious feeling of having to remember to breathe;
- the feeling of not getting enough oxygen in.

> 'Lungs that burnt and felt full of flour, making it impossible to get
> a full breath or to feel a full breath. For six months. I will NEVER
> forget that suffocating feeling. Every day and night.'

If you're exercising heavily, it is a normal physiological response to breathe harder and faster. Indeed, at a certain level of exercise, everybody will feel breathless to a degree, as increasing your breathing rate enables your body to take up more oxygen. But if you become short of breath carrying out activities you were previously doing with ease, or find your daily routine is limited due to breathing difficulties, this becomes a problem. Experiencing breathlessness can cause significant (and understandable) concern and anxiety. Breathlessness that occurs out of the blue or when you're resting can be particularly alarming.

In Long Covid, breathlessness is a commonly reported symptom. It is usual to have a degree of breathing difficulty when you are first unwell with Covid-19, but usually this resolves over a few weeks as you recover. However, if you are suffering with Long Covid, you may have found that your breathing did not improve; or it may have got better, or had never been a problem, but became an issue weeks or months down the line. It may be your main symptom and, on some days, even walking from room to room or climbing a flight of stairs can be difficult. Alternatively, breathlessness may be a relatively minor issue that waxes and wanes in the background while other symptoms, such as fatigue and brain fog, are more problematic.

It's also worth remembering that before you became unwell, exercise may have felt more difficult when you were tired or sleep deprived. The same applies to Long Covid. Many people describe feeling more breathless when their level of fatigue worsens and unpicking the two from each other can be tricky.

When we see someone with breathlessness in the clinic, we take a careful history and do a focused examination (when practical) to help determine the possible causes and decide on further management, including whether further investigations are necessary.

In our experience, people we see in the clinic who didn't require hospital admission during Covid-19 infection rarely have clinical evidence of lung or heart damage, and standard tests are typically normal. Although asthma or airways disease can sometimes flare up after having Covid, for most people this does not seem to be the explanation for their breathing problems. While we still have much to learn about what causes breathlessness, we do know that many people develop an abnormal breathing pattern (termed 'breathing pattern disorder') following Covid and this appears to heighten the sensation of breathlessness. Turn to chapter 3 for some practical ways to help manage breathlessness.

If you were admitted to hospital with Covid pneumonia, on the other hand, and particularly if you were very ill and required critical care support, follow-up tests may reveal that you have some persisting lung abnormalities. The types of investigations that are considered when evaluating people with breathlessness following Covid-19 are listed in appendix 3 at the back of the book.

Cough

A cough is a classic symptom of Covid-19 and commonly lingers for some weeks afterwards. For some people, the cough can persist beyond this. A post-viral cough following an upper respiratory tract infection (including after having had a cold, flu or Covid) is common. However, if the cough persists for over eight weeks it does need assessment by a healthcare practitioner to look for alternative or additional causes. A chest X-ray may be performed and depending on the nature of the cough, additional tests such as spirometry or lung function tests may be undertaken (see more on what these are in appendix 3). Advice to help you self-manage a chronic cough following Covid (when other causes have been evaluated or treated) is provided in chapter 3.

Sleep disturbance

Sleep disturbance is one of the most common symptoms in Long Covid. During the early stages of the illness, many people find that they need to sleep more, which is a normal physiological response to infection. While sleeping for too long can end up being an issue, more commonly people experiencing Long Covid struggle with the opposite problem. Difficulty in getting to sleep at night or staying asleep is often reported and sleep is typically fragmented and unrefreshing. Vivid dreams or nightmares can occur, particularly in those who were critically ill during their acute illness. Ways to help with sleep disturbance in Long Covid are discussed in chapter 4.

Low mood and anxiety

Many people, yourself probably included, were fit and healthy before developing Long Covid, with little in the way of pre-existing medical problems. You may have had a busy work and home life, maintaining an expertly trodden balance between the two. The symptoms of Long Covid at their worst can be such that even basic daily activities are difficult or impossible to complete. Pleasurable activities such as socialising and exercise cannot even be contemplated due to the disabling nature of fatigue and other symptoms. Employment may be affected, and you may not have been able to return to normal hours or even work at all.

The impact all this has on confidence and self-esteem can be substantial. This, coupled with a reduction in social interactions and a common feeling that others simply do not understand, can lead to a sense of isolation or loneliness. Stress can also play a major role and the understandable frustration of not getting better can negatively feed back on symptoms and hamper recovery. These issues, as well as many others induced by Long Covid, can result in low mood, anxiety or depression. The impact of Long Covid on psychological well-being is detailed in chapter 6.

*'Fatigue does not do justice to the experience. Fatigue means there is less of you. You are less. You can't, just can't, get out of bed. This is **not** psychological (although fatigue may cause depression). Your body, physically, does not have the energy.'*

Smell disturbance

'For six months after leaving hospital, I had this constant background smell. It was disgusting, it smelt like something rotting and would not go away. It put me off my food, and eating was a real struggle. Then it just faded away, I can't remember how quickly, but my smell and taste are now back to normal. Such a relief.'

Loss of smell is reported to occur in around half of people with acute Covid infection. For most people, this sense recovers relatively quickly after the initial infection. However, national data from the UK has found that almost a tenth of patients experience ongoing loss of smell several weeks after the initial infection, and in a smaller proportion this problem can persist for months, with recovery that is slow and occasionally incomplete. Our olfactory sense is responsible for picking up many of the flavours in the food we eat, so it also affects our sense of taste, and this impacts on both appetite and enjoyment of eating. Impaired smell can significantly reduce quality of life and many people we see in clinic report that this is one of the worst symptoms for them.

There are different types of smell problems following Covid. Some people find that their sense of smell is reduced (hyposmia), whereas others find that smells are altered and often unpleasant (parosmia). Less often, people report a constant background smell that is usually disagreeable and is thought to originate from within the brain (phantosmia). Commonly reported smells include burning paper, petrol and cigarette smoke. Smell disturbance and ways to aid smell recovery are covered in detail in chapter 7.

Chest pains

Chest pains are common in Long Covid and are experienced in many ways. Some people describe a 'lung burn' while for others the pain is focused around a specific area of the chest, such as between the shoulder blades, around the heart area or on one side. The pains may move around the chest and change in character. More than one type of pain can exist at the same time. The pains can be sharp, dull, tight or squeezing. They can come on gradually or suddenly, stopping people in their tracks. If you suffer with chest pains, you may find that they are more severe when other symptoms such as fatigue and breathlessness are also problematic.

Medical evaluation is important to rule out serious heart and lung conditions. Reassuringly, however, these are seldom found in people not hospitalised with Covid. Sometimes the description of chest pains enables us to work out the source of the pain (for example, a musculoskeletal problem affecting the muscles, bones or tendons, or due to inflammation around the lining of the lung). More commonly, however, the origin of these pains remains unclear and investigations do not usually provide an answer. Helpful tips to manage chest pains can be found in chapter 8.

Palpitations/rapid heart rate

Many people with Long Covid describe an increased awareness of their heartbeat (often referred to as palpitations) alongside the feeling of their heart racing (known as tachycardia). Sometimes this happens on standing up and can be associated with dizziness. These symptoms are not unique to Long Covid and are something that we see following other viral infections. Investigations such as a heart tracing (an ECG) may confirm a fast heart rate but rarely reveals other abnormalities. If you suffer with palpitations, you will know that they can be really unpleasant and cause considerable anxiety. Over time, we have come to learn that the palpitations experienced in Long Covid are almost never dangerous. Chapter 8 covers the nature and practical management of palpitations in more detail.

Dizziness

Dizziness, vertigo and imbalance symptoms usually resolve during the recovery period in the weeks following the infection, but can be a persistent or intermittent problem for some individuals with Long Covid. The reasons people struggle with ongoing dizziness are not completely understood and there may be more than one explanation in some cases. While these symptoms can also be unpleasant, they rarely indicate a serious underlying medical problem. Chapter 8 provides information to help self-manage dizziness and balance problems after having had Covid.

Gastrointestinal disturbance

Gastrointestinal symptoms such as diarrhoea, constipation, bloating and nausea have all been reported by people suffering with Long Covid. The cause of these symptoms remains unclear but they do need medical assessment in the first instance. When other explanations for these symptoms have been ruled out, there are practical measures, covered in chapter 8, that you can take to help reduce the impact of these symptoms.

Hair, nail and skin changes

Changes in hair, nails and skin are fairly common following Covid. After hospital admission in particular, many people report hair loss and nail changes. These are a recognised phenomenon following acute illness and are discussed further in chapter 8.

Fever

Intermittent fever is a recognised symptom in Long Covid and can persist for many months after the initial infection. However, it is important to note that a fever due to Long Covid is a diagnosis of exclusion, which essentially means other causes need to be ruled out first. Therefore, a thorough medical evaluation is recommended, with selected investigations including blood tests, urine tests, X-rays, and sometimes other more detailed imaging. When no other cause has been found, a fever attributed to Long Covid usually settles over several months, but occasionally can continue for more than a year.

Clinical evaluation of Long Covid

As we learn more about Long Covid, the way in which we assess and manage people at specialist centres continues to evolve. We have become skilled in recognising the major symptoms, and many of the less frequent ones too. We now realise that sophisticated investigations are often not required to confirm the diagnosis and that simple 'screening tests' may be all that are needed. One of the key roles of clinicians within the Long Covid clinic is to take a careful history and consider alternative or additional causes for symptoms. Appendix 3 lists some of the tests that may be considered if you visit your healthcare provider or attend a Long Covid clinic.

Whether you need specialist assessment or not depends to a large extent on your symptoms, and the impact your condition is having on your life. If the symptoms you experience following Covid infection are typical of Long Covid and relatively mild, it may be possible for you to self-manage at home. In fact, over time, a significant proportion of people do get better from Long Covid of their own accord, without the need for professional input.

While there is a pressing need to understand the biological drivers of Long Covid and develop better treatments, we do know that rehabilitation and management strategies, many of which were adapted from other chronic health conditions, have proved to be essential tools in setting people on the path to recovery. Much of the work we do in the Long Covid service is to equip people with the knowledge, skills and strategies to help them better manage their condition. People are recovering from Long Covid and there is light at the end of the tunnel. This book is the culmination of the work we do within the clinic and aims to provide you with tried and tested practical advice to keep you moving towards recovery.

> 'Long Covid is a terrifying and lonely journey. I've never felt so vulnerable in my life, I've sat on the end of my bed and cried more than I've cried in my life. Horrendous symptoms with no answers and no cure. It's an evil dementor in virus form.
>
> 'BUT. And it's a but, but I am getting better. It's slow but I am getting better. There are silver linings. I know my body better. I've slowed my life down. I've met many warriors and survivors and inspiring people. And I am getting better.'

'Now, I am doing a lot better. I have not had any symptoms for six weeks. What does that mean? Well, for me, it means the world. It feels like a miracle. However, otherwise, it means nothing. Doesn't mean you can ignore Long Covid.'

SUMMARY

- Long Covid is a complex condition that can affect anyone regardless of age and gender, whether you've had severe or mild Covid-19 infection.

- Symptoms are diverse and fluctuate over time, but fatigue, brain fog and breathlessness are the commonly reported problems.

- Clinical assessment in specialist services is useful for confirming the diagnosis and assisting with rehabilitation strategies, but isn't always necessary.

- We have much to learn about what causes Long Covid and as we develop a better understanding of its biological basis, specific evidence-based treatments may emerge.

- As with all chronic health conditions, a key focus of Long Covid management is providing practical advice, strategies and techniques to help you manage your symptoms while allowing time for your body to recover.

CHAPTER 2

Managing Fatigue

This chapter will take you through the fatigue management processes that we frequently use with patients attending the Long Covid clinic. The strategies are designed to help you understand your own fatigue, guiding you as you manage your activity and energy, making your life easier and supporting your recovery.

What is fatigue?

Fatigue can be such a difficult symptom to describe. It can be even more difficult to understand for those who don't have it or have never experienced it.

People struggling with chronic fatigue often say that the response they get from others if they try to tell them about their fatigue goes along the lines of 'Oh yeah, I get tired' or 'I've got that, ha ha'.

A common description is: 'It's like a heaviness' or 'I feel like I'm wading through concrete'. Others say it is like 'living with flu, day in day out'. And yet even that can seem an inadequate description for how debilitating fatigue can be.

> 'The fatigue was so difficult to cope with. People who saw me said I "looked fine" when inside I was just exhausted and felt so unwell. I could not complete a day's work and felt I was not performing. I ended up crashing and sleeping right after work to do exactly the same thing the next day.'

Everyone experiences tiredness – at the end of the day, or maybe after doing something very active or following a disturbed night. It's usually resolved by a good night's sleep, or half an hour with your feet up and a cup of tea or just a couple of days at a slower pace.

Fatigue, however, goes beyond normal tiredness and is not just a physical sensation but a cognitive (mental) thing too. It is persistent (chronic), in that it doesn't go away, no matter how much rest or sleep you have. It can be debilitating, so much so that it interferes significantly with day-to-day activities. If you have fatigue, you don't just feel exhausted or tired, but really ill.

It's important to remember that fatigue is very common after an infection and can persist for several weeks while your body recovers. However, in some cases it can stretch into several months.

Although there are no specific medications available to cure or treat the fatigue, there are many things you can do to help manage your energy levels and positively support your body's recovery. It may mean, however, that for now you might have to do things a little differently to how you've done them before.

*'Learning how to do things differently, to pace things, to acknowledge my improvement each week or month and **not** compare myself to how I was before Covid has been a huge insight. Traditionally I have pushed through colds and flu-like viruses. With Covid, I learned the hard way that this was not possible as it would lead to crashing and some symptoms returning, especially the fatigue and breathlessness.'*

A familiar symptom

While we are still gaining a greater understanding of Long Covid, we do know quite a lot about fatigue. Fatigue is a symptom of many other conditions – people who have multiple sclerosis, Parkinson's disease, hypothyroidism, and of course ME/CFS, experience fatigue as one of their main symptoms. Fatigue is also commonly seen in those recovering from infection, surgery or major medical events, such as heart attack or stroke.

The energy management approaches outlined in this chapter are used in all these situations and are techniques that you can adopt to help you recover from Long Covid.

'The important thing to remember is that the way you feel right now isn't permanent. Things do get much easier with time. I found

celebrating the little wins each day really helped to keep me motivated, no matter how small they were. Staying present in the moment is key, don't worry about how you'll feel tomorrow or in three hours' time, just focus on the moment you are in and how it serves you and your recovery.'

What's going on with your energy?

One way of thinking about fatigue is to imagine a mobile phone battery. As part of Long Covid, the battery is a lot smaller than it used to be and in not such great condition. Before you were unwell, you might have had a much larger, better-quality battery that allowed you to get through each day or week without even thinking about how much energy was in there. It recharged itself regularly and, with relaxation or a good night's sleep, would top itself up easily. However, now you will have to think about this reduced battery and consider:

- How are you going to use the energy that you do have wisely?
- How can you keep charging it up?
- How can you gradually improve the quality and size of the battery?

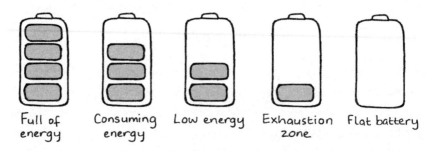

Full of energy — Consuming energy — Low energy — Exhaustion zone — Flat battery

The 3 Ps: Prioritising – Planning – Pacing

The 3 Ps can be a very useful way to start thinking about managing your fatigue and it's useful to keep these principles in mind throughout the chapter.

Prioritising

When any of us experience a health condition, it is often useful to re-examine priorities and consider if any might need adjusting. Thinking about that battery, and the fact that it is not quite so big now: are there any areas in your life where you might be able to conserve some energy? Why waste the energy that you do have? Save some for the things that are important and meaningful to you.

Switches or changes you could consider might include:

- doing an online shop rather than going to the supermarket;
- taking the bus rather than walking to work;
- accepting help with chores around the house when offered.

'Take the help, from anyone who offers, and drop the guilt that comes with saying "no" to things. The people who matter the most will still be there at the end of the day and allowing them to help you lets them feel useful as well, it must be very hard for our families to see us so poorly and not be able to fix it for us. Seeing their happiness in helping you will give you a boost as well, you can feel the love and support, which creates a safe space for healing.'

To help with this, you could ask yourself the following questions:

- What must get done?
- What can wait?
- What really isn't necessary?
- What can be scrubbed off the list entirely?
- What can be done by someone else?
- What would I really like to be doing with my energy and time?

As part of this, you might want to consider if you are putting yourself under any undue pressure. If you are someone who has high standards or particular ways of doing things, you may find the chapter on psychological aspects of Long Covid helpful.

'Outsource whatever you can afford and feel comfortable doing. If it's not possible, be kind and forgiving to yourself. If you can't change your bedsheets this month – it's fine. If you have to buy frozen meals, it's also fine. You are only accountable for yourself, not what others think.'

Planning

Planning how you are going to spend your day and carry out your activities can be really helpful in managing the energy you do have in your battery. This applies to both large events and tasks and the smaller things you do.

Some examples to consider:

- If you find medical appointments demanding, could you build in some recovery time afterwards?
- Could you arrange that important phone call or work meeting for a time in the day where you usually feel better?
- If you have a bit more energy in the evening, could you shower then rather than in the morning?
- If you tend to tire by the afternoon, is it possible to set aside some time to rest and do a relaxation exercise earlier in the day to allow you to have more energy later on?
- If you are cooking, could you batch cook and freeze some?
- If you like to go shopping – could you plan to go to just one or two shops and then come home and rest?
- Could you attend that social event – just for an hour?
- Could a friend or family member drive you to an event?

Pacing

You might have heard of pacing as a technique but don't really know what it means in practice.

Generally, it's about doing things at a level lower than your maximum capacity to ensure you have enough energy for an activity or activities. Sports people use it all the time to optimise their energy use. A pacer in a big race will support runners or cyclists to stick to the speed necessary to maintain stamina and to eliminate the problem of accidentally over-extending themselves and having to drop out of the race, exhausted. You might remember the Aesop fable about the tortoise and the hare: it was the tortoise who won the race, not the speedy hare, the moral being that you can be more successful by doing things slowly and steadily than by acting quickly and carelessly.

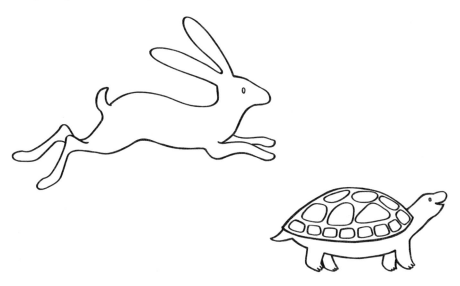

'I found real comfort in slowing down. I've always been a very busy person and often didn't take the time to stop and appreciate things around me. Long Covid forced me to slow down, to stop and look and feel the world around me differently. It's actually quite beautiful when you have the time to absorb it fully. I will remember to take those moments still when I'm fully recovered, it's very humbling to feel this grateful to still be here.'

However, when we look at energy management overall, it's not just about pacing an activity, it's a broader concept. It's about creating a balance between activity and rest.

In practical terms, this generally means doing a little something then having a rest, doing a little something, then having a rest. In the past, you might have been able to go from job to job throughout the day, lie on the sofa in the evening, go to bed and then get up the next morning with your energy battery topped up and ready to do the same thing again. But because your battery is smaller right now, you will need to keep topping it up regularly throughout the day. It may be that you will need to break that activity down into even smaller chunks, so rather than vacuuming the whole house in one go and then sitting down for a cup of tea, you might need to do just one room and then rest. You may even find that vacuuming isn't possible at the moment, in which case, see 'prioritising' (p. 27) and consider accepting help with housework, even if it isn't up your usual standards.

Pacing applies to cognitive (mental) tasks too – these use just as much energy from the battery. So rather than sitting and working at the computer for two hours, you may need to stop after 30 minutes and rest. Some people find it helpful to set an alarm as a reminder to pause for five minutes on the hour, every hour.

If you can, mix up cognitive and physical tasks throughout the day. This takes less of a toll on the battery. Big chunks of physical or cognitive activity can significantly drain your resources.

Knowing when to stop
You may never have had to consider your stopping point before. When your battery was much bigger, there was always enough in there to get you through the day. The lack of energy can feel very frustrating and over-whelming at times, especially when there are things you want or need to be doing. However, as part of pacing, it's helpful to consider when and how you are going to stop so that you avoid flattening that battery. You will know from experience that if your mobile phone completely flattens, you can't do anything with it until it's recharged to a certain point. If you can keep topping up your own energy regularly before it gets flat, there is always some available for you to do things.

Listening to your body and observing how it responds to activity is a useful first step in learning when it might be appropriate to stop or where to set the limits. You may notice that you have a fairly immediate response to overdoing an activity, in that you feel tired or lose energy part way through. Or you may have a delayed reaction – you feel all right at the time but later that day, or the next, you feel flooded with exhaustion. This is known as post-exertional malaise. It may be easy to overlook your body's warning signals, but over time you can learn to avoid overdoing things that flatten the battery and lead to post-exertional malaise.

Understanding this process and drawing on what you know from your responses can help you to develop reliable ways of stopping and resting early enough, such as establishing time limits or task limits. For example, if you have learned from experience that after 10 minutes of reading your concentration and focus reduces and you struggle to take in and retain the words, feeling that your brain is foggy, you know you will need to stop at this point and not push through. Or if you know that a day of gardening will wipe you out for the next two days, you could set yourself the task of tidying up just one small section and then stop for the day.

By **chunking** activities, breaking them down into smaller chunks by either time or activity and being clear on the stopping point, you can reserve some energy so there is always a little bit spare, should you need it.

Some useful principles of pacing:

- Do a little something then rest, do a little something then rest.
- Mix up cognitive and physical tasks throughout the day and intersperse with periods of rest.
- 'Chunk' activity – break things down into smaller, more manageable chunks.
- Set the limit or end point before you start – it's easy to get carried away in the moment.
- Use an alarm to remind you to stop.
- Slow down – be a tortoise!

'Trust the process and don't fight your own body. Really learn to listen to your body. It's all about learning what works for you. Once I started really becoming the observer to my own body I could respond more appropriately with what it needed.'

Rest

We've established that for now it's important to pace yourself and balance your physical and mental activity with periods of rest. But what is rest? It can mean different things to different people and can often be misunderstood, or not taken seriously enough. Some people seem to be very good at rest, whereas others find it difficult to stop or even see the value in rest.

Here's a couple of definitions of rest:

- 'Cease work or movement in order to relax, sleep or recover strength'
- 'Allow to be inactive in order to regain strength or health'*

It's a good idea to think about the difference between rest and low-level activity. Many of us *think* we are resting when in fact we are engaging in a low-level activity. Reading a book or a magazine, watching TV, scrolling through our phone: these are low-level activities, and while they do not require a huge amount of energy (and are good to do in your day), they are still using up a little. Proper, restorative/healing rest helps to put some energy into your battery – to charge it up. Rests are 'pauses' of activity. These might be in the form of relaxation exercises, breathing exercises, meditation techniques, mindfulness, restorative yoga practice or soothing sensory techniques such as sound apps, a heated blanket, or aromatherapy. Find a way of *truly* resting that works for you. It's best if you can rest away from your bedroom so you can keep the bedroom just for sleep.

Many people express feelings of guilt about stopping and resting or view it as a negative thing. This can act as a barrier to resting. If this sounds famil-iar, try to reframe your attitude to rest in a positive light. By resting you are not doing nothing, you are recharging your battery. You will be doing your-self (and those around you) a huge favour.

> 'After looking at my day more closely, I realised that I wasn't resting very much at all. I was worried that if I stopped I wouldn't be able to get started again. I was encouraged to give it a go and see what happened. I planned in regular, only short, rest intervals throughout my day, and I found that I could cope with my day a lot better.'

Is sleep a restful activity?

Sometimes, sleep and rest are used interchangeably (*see* the first definition above). However, in terms of health, they are different and play different roles in our well-being.

Sleep is essential for survival. Sleep loss over time can lead to health

---

* Definitions taken from *Oxford Languages* (Google's English dictionary).

problems and directly impacts on almost every bodily system. Rest does not involve quite the same level of disengagement as sleep and is often defined as a behaviour designed to increase physical and mental well-being.

Both sleep and rest are essential and while rest can be simply a useful opportunity to hit the pause button, it can also pave the way to a better night's sleep. Many people describe a 'tired but wired' feeling at night, often making it difficult to get to sleep or to have a restful sleep. Engaging in regular rest throughout the day can help to avoid this feeling.

'Try to find things that help you feel calm, happy and safe. You need to get rid of the fight or flight mode that comes from severe illness, trauma and running on empty, and instead practise deep, conscious rest and restorative experiences that promote healing.'

However, try to avoid napping during the day if you can, as this can affect your sleep at night. If you need to nap, or think you might fall asleep while resting, set an alarm so you do not nap for long (there is more detailed information about this in chapter 4, Sleep and Long Covid).

Where do I start with managing the fatigue?

There is a series of steps we go through at the clinic with people experiencing fatigue. This is predominantly around how to manage activity and rest. It's worth saying here that it is not always a linear process, and everyone is different, so we might move back and forth between the steps set out below until we find the right balance.

Finding the baseline

Figuring out your baseline is an important first step towards managing fatigue and supporting your recovery journey. Your baseline is the level of activity that you can manage, day-to-day, without making your fatigue and other symptoms worse. The idea is that it can help you to stabilise your energy levels, lay the foundations and allow you to create a stable platform on which to build your energy and activity levels over time.

First, you need to look at what is happening now: with your symptoms, what you are doing, what choices you are making and what patterns may be forming, some of which may be helping and others that may be less helpful in the long run. The steps that follow can help with this process.

STEP ONE: Understanding patterns

Boom and bust

One of the patterns that can commonly occur with fatigue and a smaller battery is the 'boom and bust'. You may find that your fatigue levels fluctuate – you might have a day where you feel you have a little more energy than usual, so you rush round getting everything done that you haven't managed to get to for days or weeks. Unfortunately, there isn't that amount of energy in your battery right now to cope with this and you can end up 'crashing'. A crash is an increase in symptoms, and you may find you need to rest more as a result. The crash may last days or even weeks.

A degree of boom and bust can happen in normal life. Life gets busy at times, and with a bigger and better functioning battery the crashes are not so devastating and debilitating. A good night's sleep or a quieter day and things soon feel back to normal. However, when you have a smaller battery, this pattern can prolong the fatigue and over time your capacity to do things becomes less and less, thus slowing down recovery (*see* graph 1).

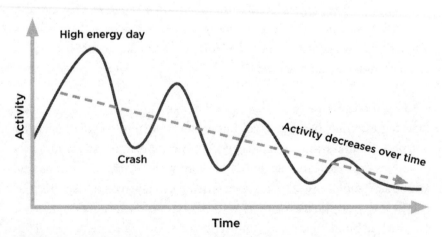

GRAPH 1: Boom and bust.

Avoiding

Sometimes, because of the boom and bust or unpleasant increases in symptoms, or even the constant day-to-day struggle, you might start to limit activities more and more or avoid them altogether. This may be driven by a fear of making things worse or an attempt to make them better. Worries and stress can start to creep in and you can end up in a vicious cycle. This is completely understandable; you will do anything to avoid the potential to make things worse and to minimise any worry or stress. Significantly restricting or avoiding means you are no longer falling into the boom-and-bust trap, but unfortunately it can lead to things getting rather stuck and the battery failing to charge. The human battery needs an element of activity to produce energy. By limiting or avoiding activity and resting too much, you can feel more lethargic and increase symptoms such as pain and stiffness. It can also impact on your concentration, memory and brain fog, and not least your mood and emotional health. That's not to say rest isn't good – it is – but it's finding the right level for the stage that you're at (*see* graph 2).

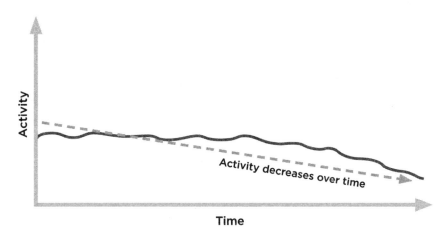

GRAPH 2: Avoiding activity.

Pushing through

Some people try to push through the fatigue or to do things as they did before they were unwell. You might be trying to force yourself through your list of tasks even though you feel exhausted, or maybe you were the sort of person who previously could go from job to job throughout the day, barely stopping, and that's what you're continuing to do now.

Unfortunately, thinking about that battery size, you haven't the energy in there to cope with that at the moment. The body, however, will often try to adapt, and may attempt to use adrenaline as backup. While adrenaline is important in the body – it prepares you for the fight and flight response (an automatic physiological reaction to an event that is perceived as stressful or frightening) – overusing it can have a negative impact. Repeatedly relying on your body's reserves when your battery is in the exhaustion zone can again make the fatigue worse or last longer, like the boom and bust approach (*see* graph 1).

> *'Acceptance on how you are and feel right now and letting go of the anger/grief about how you used to feel and behave is key to recovering. Once you get to a peaceful state of acceptance and can be kind to yourself, you are on to a winner.'*

How are you using the energy that you have in your battery? Are you booming and busting? Are you worried about doing anything in case you make it worse or are you trying to ignore the fatigue and push through? Whatever your pattern, these responses are very common and familiar to those experiencing fatigue. To understand this more fully, it's helpful to monitor your energy expenditure throughout the day and across the week. You may begin to notice patterns in your energy consumption and how you are undertaking activity (*see* step 4). But first it's useful to go through step 2.

STEP TWO: Understanding energy requirements for activities

Some activities will take a lot of energy from the battery, others a little less and some just a small amount. We label these as high-, medium- and low-energy expenditure. Take some time to work out what you do each day, and include both the physical and mental tasks. Consider also any emotional or stressful issues as part of this analysis. Stress (which can be a part of everyday life and is often a factor when dealing with a health issue) is greedy and can take a considerable amount of energy from the battery. Use the energy requirements form to start making your list. You can add to it as you go about your week.

These energy requirements will be unique to you and the stage you are at in your recovery. What one person finds requires a high level of energy, another person may find requires only a medium amount of energy.

Energy requirements form

Low (Green)	Medium (Yellow)	High (Red)
e.g. Reading a novel/ watching TV	e.g. Driving locally/ familiar trip	e.g. Tricky meeting with work
e.g. Brushing teeth	e.g. Getting dressed	e.g. Showering

Many people think, because of the fatigue and reduced energy levels, that they are not doing anything with their day – they are comparing themselves to what they were like and what they did before. Remember, everything you do, even if it feels like it is less than before, is still an activity. Getting up and dressed is an activity, getting breakfast is an activity, sending an email is an activity. All of these are achievements throughout the day. They may be small but they are definitely significant.

STEP THREE:
Understanding your supply and demand

Keeping with the battery idea, there will be various things throughout the day that take energy from the battery, and some activities will take more energy than others. But there will also be things that can give you energy. There are the more obvious factors such as sleep, food, hydration and rest, but things that are fun or pleasurable or give you a sense of satisfaction can also help recharge the battery. Again, these will be unique to you in terms of what you find meaningful or enjoyable. It might include time with friends, preparing a nice dinner, or engaging in a particular hobby that you have.

Have a think about your own personal supply and demand and add to the list below:

Supply and demand form

Things that take my energy:
i.e.
❏ Work
❏ Showering
❏ Stress
❏ ....
❏ ....
❏ ....
❏ ....
❏ ....
❏ ....
❏ ....

Things that give me energy:
i.e.
❏ Sleep
❏ Healthy food
❏ Rest
❏ ....
❏ ....
❏ ....
❏ ....
❏ ....
❏ ....
❏ ....

'I made a list of things on my phone that were easy to do and would bring me joy. They would give me a lift and act as a little bit of a spark. To me, tending to low-maintenance houseplants was just great. Lighting scented candles and using nice soaps or hand creams was also great. Flicking through gardening and interior magazines was lovely and didn't require too much concentration. I even rearranged some small things around my house, changed my scenery a bit.'

STEP FOUR: Energy expenditure

Once you have begun to understand the things that give you energy – and how much energy things take – you can begin to understand how you are 'spending' that energy. If you're a person who finds it easier to think visually, then you might want to have a go at the energy map overleaf. This allows you to plot how you do things over a fortnightly period and you can see very quickly what patterns have been forming. For example, the map can show if you have big clusters of high-level activity that might be causing a 'crash' after a few days. As this book is in black and white, we've used patterns to indicate the different levels of activity, but you could use colour – for example, low activity = green, medium = yellow, high = red, rest = purple, sleep = blue.

What we're aiming for over time, where possible, is a reasonable balance of low, medium and high levels of activity across the day/week.

You may prefer to keep an activity diary, which can contain a bit more detail, and rate your levels of fatigue following the activity alongside. An example of this follows, together with a blank template and a less detailed version.

Figure out which version works best for you – the purpose of the exercise is to understand where and how you have been spending your energy, to identify any patterns and help you work out your baseline.

'To me, fatigue is like having an energy bank account. It's an account where I have suddenly lost lots of money, so I have less to play with and I need to be careful what I spend it on. I start the day with 100 energy coins in my account: getting out of bed is two

coins, getting dressed – three, making breakfast – five coins and so on. I can use more coins than I have, but then I would need to dip into my overdraft and have to pay my debt with high interest over the next few days. I can earn more coins and top up my account with rest periods and use fewer coins if I pace my activities.'

Energy Map

Week 1 (/ /20)																									
	Morning (AM)												Afternoon (PM)												
	12-1am	1	2	3	4	5	6	7	8	9	10	11	12	1	2	3	4	5	6	7	8	9	10	11
Mon																								
Tue																								
Wed																								
Thu																								
Fri																								
Sat																								
Sun																								

Week 2 (/ /20)																									
	Morning (AM)												Afternoon (PM)												
	12-1am	1	2	3	4	5	6	7	8	9	10	11	12	1	2	3	4	5	6	7	8	9	10	11
Mon																								
Tue																								
Wed																								
Thu																								
Fri																								
Sat																								
Sun																								

KEY

High energy activity

Medium energy activity

Low energy activity

Rest / Chillout time

Sleep

Activity diary (option 1, example)
Day 1

Time	Activity	Fatigue rating 0 = low 10 = high
8:30 – 8:45	Up and showered	7
8:45 – 9:00	Dressed	8
9:00 – 9:15	Breakfast	7
9:15 – 9:30	Rest	3
9:30 – 9:40	Put a wash on	4
9:40 – 10:00	Phoned a friend	5
10:00 – 10:30	Read my book	4
10:30 – 10:45	Hung the washing out	8
10:45 – 11:00	Caught up on emails	6
11:00 – 11:15	Cleared up the kitchen	5
11:15 – 12:00	Watched TV with cup of tea	4
12:00 – 12:30	Had lunch	6
12:30 – 13:30	Went for a walk	9
13:30 – 14:00	Rest	4
14:00 – 14:30	Drove to the supermarket	9
14:30 – 15:30	Supermarket shop	10
15:30 – 16:00	Drove home	10
16:00 – 16:30	Put food away	9
16:30 – 17:00	Started food prep	9
17:00 – 18:15	Rest – fell asleep	7
18:15 – 19:00	Cooked	8
19:00 – 19:30	Ate dinner	7
19:30 – 19:50	Cleared up the kitchen	9
19:50 – 21:00	Watched TV	6
21:00 – 21:30	Bedtime prep/read	5
21:45	Asleep	

Activity Diary (option 1)
Day 1

Time	Activity	Fatigue rating 0 = low 10 = high

Activity Diary (option 2)
Week 1

Time	Mon	Tue	Wed	Thu	Fri	Sat	Sun
8:00 – 9:00							
9:00 – 10:00							
10:00 – 11:00							
11:00 – 12:00							
12:00 – 13:00							
13:00 – 14:00							
14:00 – 15:00							
15:00 – 16:00							
16:00 – 17:00							
17:00 – 18:00							
18:00 – 19:00							
19:00 – 20:00							
20:00 – 21:00							
21:00 – 22:00							
22:00 – 00:00							
Went to sleep							

These steps can help you to understand what is happening and stabilise your energy levels much as possible. It's sometimes referred to as 'zooming out'. It can help you to avoid those less helpful 'boom and bust' patterns, doing too little or pushing through. You can begin to understand where your energy goes and what gives you energy. It can provide you with insight as to where you might need to rest more or do a little less and where to implement the Prioritising, Planning, Pacing (3Ps) – thus creating a more stable platform. It allows you to gain more control and provide a firmer foundation from which to build. We call this a baseline.

'I've learnt to be aware of my own energy resources each day, working out how I use them, both in work, at home and socially meeting up with friends and family. All of this takes energy. Keeping a diary made me realise when I had done too much and how it affected me. I could then adjust to how I did things. Currently doing things for smaller amounts of time during the day, stopping in the evenings and going to bed earlier works for me. It is important to find what works for you. I still do not yet have the energy levels that I had before Covid but managing my energy during the day and putting into place breathing exercises and mindfulness sessions is helping me move forward with my recovery. I am reminding myself that each day is often a little bit better, sometimes I crash but I am slowly moving forward on the scale, accepting what is and knowing that I am getting there.'

Setting the baseline

In the graph opposite, you can see that stabilisation doesn't mean a completely flat line of steady activity – this would just not be possible. But keeping your activities within a manageable range for you is what you're aiming for. Your fatigue levels will still fluctuate to a certain degree but by avoiding excessive over- or under-activity, you can find a balance and start to build your energy and activity levels over time.

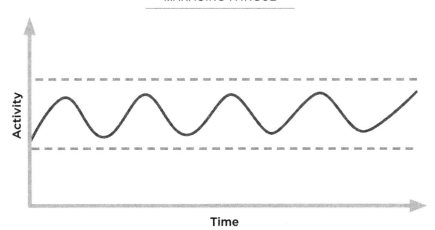

GRAPH 3: Stabilisation.

TIPS FOR SETTING YOUR BASELINE

- Sometimes you might be a little overambitious and set the baseline too high, doing too much. Cut it down to 75 per cent or even 50 per cent, to where you think it might need to be. It doesn't matter how small it is at this stage, it's about stabilisation.
- The aim of a baseline of activity is a level that you can manage on both a good and a bad day – not exceeding it on a good day.
- Try using an activity planner or one of the diary templates in this chapter that stretch across the day or week to help you prioritise and pace your activities. This can be especially helpful if you are experiencing brain fog (see chapter 8). Written plans can provide you with a useful reminder of what activities and tasks are required for the week, giving you less to think about, rather than trying to hold it all in your head.
- Life may intervene in your plans and get in the way – that's OK – **be flexible with your plan**. If you are implementing the 3Ps principle (Prioritise – what is important and what can wait, Planning – think ahead to spread out the energy usage, Pacing – take it slow and give yourself permission to take those rests), there may well be a little bit of energy in the battery to cope with any changes. If not, plan in some recovery time.

TIP

Finding your baseline can be a process of experimentation and your baseline will be different to someone else's. You might not get it right straight away, and although it can be extremely frustrating, it's totally normal. Use the information as feedback and adjust accordingly. Some people like to use diaries to help plan out the week, others like to do a snapshot of the energy map every now and again just to review what's happening.

'Over time I learnt not to get too obsessed or rigid with the techniques. Initially I spent some time understanding all the essentials such as pacing, prioritising, planning etc. and getting to know my body battery well. However, it can be very overwhelming to write down every symptom and every activity all day every day for your entire journey. It will become second nature, so trust that you are learning from your experiences and focus more on the effect that happy/positive experiences have on how you feel and what improvements you are seeing.'

Pacing up

Finding the baseline is a key part of the recovery journey. As we have seen, it can take quite a bit of time and tweaking, trial and error, and establishing that baseline may be all you need to do for this stage of your recovery.

However, once things have stabilised, and you have become much more familiar with and expert at using the 3Ps (Prioritising – Planning – Pacing), you might feel ready or wish to consider a pacing-up approach.

Pacing up is a careful and considered approach to increasing activity, not necessarily involving exercise. You might have read some of the conflicting information about graded exercise or GET (graded exercise therapy) in relation to chronic fatigue and it might be useful to stress at this point that pacing up is not GET.

Pacing up will be unique to you and the level of your own baseline, but there is a process to help guide you. Start with adding in just one new activity or lengthening an existing one. It could be either a physical or a cognitive (mental) activity.

The analogy of a staircase is often used, as opposed to a slope; each level or stair is a very small step up and needs to be maintained before the next step is taken. For example, rather than increasing a daily walk each time you go out, keep it at this level for a week or two and then consider the next increase, depending on how you feel.

If you are more severely affected and feel you are at the stage where you could begin to pace up an activity, this might mean, for example, listening to the radio for a bit longer or having longer conversations with people.

Keep the increase very small, so it will have minimal impact on your body. We often suggest around 10 per cent more initially. It's better to take smaller steps and be successful than to take one big step and end up crashing (and back in that boom and bust). As time goes on, and if you are finding that your body is getting stronger, you may be able to make slightly bigger increases – figure out what works for you.

As you make the increase, you may notice a slight and temporary increase in sensations, such as stiffness, fatigue or brain fog. This is normal and to be expected and will hopefully settle quickly after a day or even a few hours. However, if the sensations persist for a week or more, it may mean that the increase was too much or too quick. Adjust it accordingly.

KEY POINT
It's important to give your body the time to settle at its baseline for a while before considering a pacing-up approach.

Getting stuck

People sometimes report getting a bit stuck at a particular level with their energy management (we often refer to this as 'plateauing'). If this happens, it can be quite helpful to take an overview, work out if anything else is going on, perhaps zoom out and re-examine your energy expenditure. Have you stopped taking rests? Are you going back to old habits and doing things the way you did them before? Or maybe there are other factors that are impeding progress, some of which are explored in other chapters. It may be that this is the level where things need to be right now and that's OK for this phase of your recovery.

> 'I would say that I'm recovering. The biggest thing for me has been to accept where I am at each stage of my recovery. It's probably what helped me most early on. It's not easy and I have to make a conscious effort not to think about or compare myself to what I used to be able to do or what other people can do. I now don't worry about the future and say to myself. "Just because I am like this today, doesn't mean I'm going to be like this next year" and in fact I am getting better.'

Dealing with flare-ups and setbacks

We know that Long Covid has a fluctuating nature. Recovery is not a smooth line and it can on occasions feel like you are taking two steps forward and one step back (see graph 4 below). This can feel incredibly frustrating. Sometimes there are clear reasons as to why a flare-up or setback has occurred – it might be that you've had an exceptionally busy time, you've had another bug or virus, or things have got a bit stressful – as they do at times in life. Take some time to review what might be going on. Zoom out again. You may need to shift things down a notch or two for a short time, allow your body to recover and then pace up again slowly.

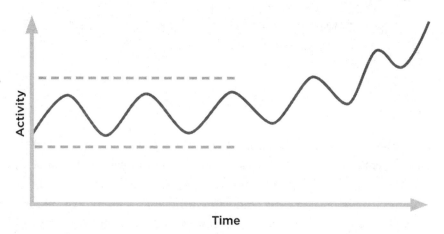

GRAPH 4: Recovery.

'Reframing how I felt when the symptoms flared up was helpful. I found that if I disassociated from them a bit, as if I was looking at myself from across the room, then I didn't feel so burdened or upset by them. Your symptoms don't define you. If you can feel them and acknowledge them without letting them overwhelm you, then you can learn to respond to them more positively.'

A's story:
'Covid brought a deep-seated fatigue that felt like I had been on the longest plane journey with the worst jet lag that didn't improve with what I thought of as "rest" and usual sleep. I had never had a problem with sleep before and usually woke up early full of energy, but sleep was no longer easy or restorative. My thinking brain felt like it had turned to custard with a difficulty in finding words, of thinking clearly, but it also felt wired and busy. I tried to push through, but that just made the extreme tiredness (both body and mind) and the other symptoms of tachycardia and headaches even worse, sometimes on the same day, sometimes days after. I learnt this was called post-exertional symptom exacerbation/malaise.

'My Long Covid occupational therapist advised me to list my daily activities into low/medium/high energy activities and suggested I complete an activity diary over a few weeks so I could see the patterns of activities and where my energy was perhaps going. I thought I was pacing my day, but the activity diary using colours for different activities hour by hour gave a visual description of how much high-energy activity I had been using without realising. Most of the day was high energy with very few rest periods. I thought rest was watching a film, scrolling on Instagram, reading a magazine, but I found this did not restore energy but used it. The diary also showed me that I was going to bed at different times of day, often quite late.

'I learnt about deep conscious rest and the importance of setting time aside for this. Gentle restorative yoga online soothed my busy body and mind, focusing on calming the breath with slow abdominal breathing and stretching out tense, sore muscles. I started regular meditation and I learnt about mindfulness, both teaching me to be in the moment, letting worrying thoughts regarding my health or tasks undone to float by, leading to a stillness of body and mind.

'Attending to a better sleep pattern was key, with the aim of getting off to sleep in a timely way, staying asleep and for sleep to bring energy for the day ahead. Blue filters on the laptop and mobile phone helped with light sensitivity and energy, but I also became mindful of not looking at or scrolling screens for an hour or two before bedtime. I stopped watching 'excitable' TV pre bedtime and tried to go to bed at the same time every night, listening to gentle wind-down classical music and meditations for sleep.

'Pacing enabled me to stop the boom and bust cycle I had been in. I started to pace, plan ahead and prioritise activities. I used a detailed diary to plan the week to ensure I had rest periods/days between activities like shopping, baking a cake or going for a drink with friends. Everyday activities were broken into chunks, for example I no longer "washed up" but used the dishwasher, unloading top shelf, then rest, then bottom shelf. I planned meals ahead, sat down to peel the veg or to mix ingredients and batch cooked and froze meals, so I'd have meals for the days where I lacked energy. Sitting down to dry myself and get dressed after a shower eased the fatigue. Switching between deep rest, cognitive activities such as answering emails/managing bills with a more body-exertional activity such as weeding the garden helped. Spreading activities over the week has now become instinctive.

'Accepting this was a 'new for now' normal, losing the fear of "What if I…?", reframing negative thoughts such as "But I used to be able…" to "If I do this, I can" has helped me progress and re-engage with joyful activities. Knowing I have the tools to manage the unpredictable days and the dips or hiccoughs that just happen in life is managing my fatigue and aiding recovery.'

SUMMARY

- Plan how you are going to do your activity and when you are going to do it.

- Set the limit before you start.

- Chunk activities – break them down into smaller, more manageable tasks.

- Make sure your rest is 'proper' rest, not a low-level activity.

- Top up your battery regularly throughout the day with 'fuel' – i.e. food and water.

- See if you can keep a little bit of energy in your battery (we all know that a flat battery means a blank screen and you can do nothing with it).

- Don't waste energy on unnecessary things – conserve it where you can. Ask for help, pay for help if you can afford it or be ruthless with your to-do list.

- Mix things up – mix up cognitive and physical activities and intersperse with rest.

- Make sure you build in those fun and pleasurable activities.

- Be kind to yourself – remember, it's the tortoise who won the race.

CHAPTER 3
Managing breathlessness

We often do not appreciate the importance of the *breath*, yet breathlessness can be one of the most distressing symptoms experienced by people suffering with Long Covid. In this chapter, we will help you to understand the power of the breath in your Long Covid recovery, as well as explore the factors that may be contributing to your breathlessness and provide you with strategies to help you control and manage it.

How Covid might affect breathing

Breathlessness is a really common symptom in Long Covid. There may be more than one reason for breathing problems after Covid and so to get a better understanding of this, it is important to consider your Covid journey and the details of your initial illness.

If you were admitted to hospital, particularly if you required a high concentration of oxygen or additional respiratory support (*see* table 3), you may have developed a degree of lung damage. Your muscles may also be weaker as a result of being severely unwell and not being able to do physical activity (we call this 'deconditioning'). This may affect your breathing and even gentle exertion in the first few months after leaving hospital may leave you struggling for breath. If you have a pre-existing lung or heart condition, having Covid may cause it to flare up, and your breathing may feel worse as a result.

Many people with Long Covid did not require hospital admission during their initial infection and do not have a history of lung or heart disease, yet also struggle with ongoing breathlessness. In this situation, we typically find that the standard tests designed to look for recognised lung and heart problems are normal. While we still have much to learn about what might be driving this sort of breathlessness, we often observe irregularities in the way that people with Long Covid breathe. We find that many people develop an altered breathing pattern that often amplifies the sensation of feeling breathless. This is most commonly referred to as a breathing pattern disorder or dysfunctional breathing.

Whether you have a recognised respiratory diagnosis or not, the strategies and advice about how you can manage and improve the burden of breathlessness are similar.

The table below shows some of the respiratory supports that you or a loved one may have experienced if you were hospitalised with Covid-19.

Types of acute inpatient respiratory support in Covid-19
Standard oxygen therapy: given via face mask or nasal cannula
High-flow oxygen therapy: oxygen therapy delivered at high flow and high concentration via nasal cushions
CPAP (continuous positive airways pressure) therapy: a tight-fitting face mask, commonly fitted over the nose and mouth, that provides increased pressure into the lungs, helping to keep airways open and improve the delivery of oxygen
Mechanical (or invasive) ventilation: a tube is inserted into the airway (the trachea) and a machine (a ventilator) supports or takes over breathing; undertaken in intensive care

TABLE 3: Types of acute inpatient respiratory support in Covid-19.

What is normal breathing?

Breathing is a completely natural, automatic and fundamental function of the human body. In simple terms, when you breathe in (inspiration), your lungs expand and fill with air. You absorb the oxygen in the air through the lining of the lungs, and it is then taken up by the blood and transported around the body. When you breathe out (expiration), you are expelling air rich in the waste gas carbon dioxide. This process is essential for the healthy functioning of the organs and cells within your body.

The process of breathing involves specific muscles that enable the lungs to fill and empty with air efficiently during rest and exercise. The main muscles involved in breathing are:

- the diaphragm
- the accessory muscles

Diaphragm

This is the dome-shaped muscle that sits at the bottom of the lungs. As you breathe in, this muscle contracts and flattens, and by doing so, it increases the space within the chest cavity to create a suction that causes the lungs to expand with air. As you breathe out, the diaphragm relaxes and returns to its dome shape, squeezing the lungs and helping expel the air. This process happens automatically and is passive, meaning that you have little control over it.

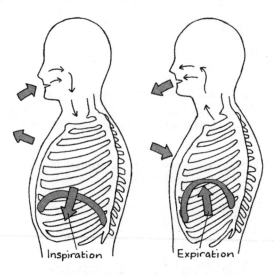

Inspiration   Expiration

DIAGRAM 1: The diaphragm and intercostal muscles are the main muscles involved in breathing.

The diaphragm can be thought of as the 'Mo Farah' of muscles. It is an endurance muscle and requires very little energy to perform.

Accessory muscles

These are a group of muscles that support the movement of the chest wall. When the muscles in between the ribs (the external intercostal muscles) contract, they expand the ribcage outwards and cause you to breathe in. When you breathe out, they relax passively. During more strenuous activity, you require more oxygen as the muscles and other tissues in the body become more active. To increase oxygen uptake, you have to breathe harder and faster. You thus start to use the additional accessory muscles that surround the chest. These muscles assist in the expansion and contraction of the ribcage, resulting in the greater movement of air in and out of the lungs.

The accessory muscles can be thought of as the 'Usain Bolts' – short sharp sprinters, using up to 30 per cent more of your body's energy to work.

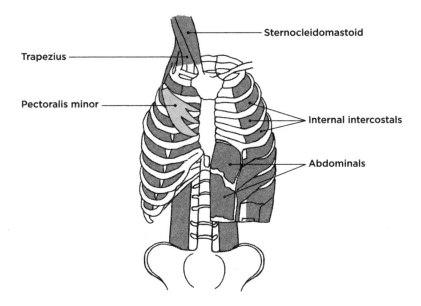

DIAGRAM 2: The accessory muscles of breathing.

During the acute phase of many illnesses, the breathing rate increases to meet the body's higher metabolic demands needed to fight infection. Additionally, respiratory infections such as Covid-19 can result in acute lung damage that may compromise function and reduce the efficiency of oxygen uptake into the body. So, the breathing rate adjusts to compensate for the decreased efficiency of the lungs, which is a normal physiological response. Similar to when exercising, this is achieved by breathing faster and using the accessory muscles. The breathing may become more shallow than usual, meaning you are breathing using the upper chest, and you often start to breathe through your mouth instead of your nose. Stress hormones associated with fight/flight (stress) responses are increased, which enhances this process. This release of adrenaline can make you feel somewhat panicky, once again speeding up the breathing rate.

Once the infection has cleared, the body usually returns to a normal state. However, we find that sometimes people appear to be stuck in this now unhelpful state and the breathing pattern that developed during the acute illness does not go away, or may do so but later returns, and can then become habitual. Switching it off can be difficult.

Bloated stomach

Palpitations

Wheeze

Dry cough

Fast and shallow breathing

Chest pain

Noisy breathing

Forgetting to breathe

Dizziness

Chest tightness

Tingling around lips

Cold hands and feet

Inability to take a deep enough breathe

Blurred vision

Air hunger

Frequent sighing or yawning

Awareness of breathing feeling unnatural

Unsatisfying breaths

Heaviness on chest

TABLE 4: Some of the symptoms often associated with breathlessness.

Breathing more than your body actually needs (or 'overbreathing') can make you feel tired and increase levels of fatigue and anxiety. The body responds automatically to feelings of anxiety by releasing stress hormones that drive the fight or flight response, resulting in a vicious cycle that worsens breathlessness and drives anxiety.

So, while your breathing pattern may not be the only reason you are experiencing these and other symptoms, it can certainly be a contributing factor.

'I used to play the flute and loved swimming, both needing good breath control: I trusted my breath. But I started to realise that speaking on the phone or on Zoom calls took huge amounts of energy and I was needing to take a quick gasp mid-sentence. Walking and talking was impossible, even walking alone seemed hard and I realised I felt breathless.'

Feeling breathless can be scary, especially when it is out of proportion to the activity you are performing. People often report feeling out of control when they can't catch their breath, but however your breathlessness affects you, learning good techniques to help you to gain control of your breathing will help.

COSTOCHONDRITIS

Many people experience pain over the centre of the chest, where the sternum (breastbone) sits. It can often feel tender to touch. For many, this causes concern due to the nature of the pain and its position near the heart. This pain is caused by irritation of the cartilage that sits between the ribs and sternum, referred to as the costochondral junctions. These can be aggravated by abnormal breathing and the friction can cause inflammation at these joints, termed costochondritis. As you begin to address any breathing issues you may have, this often settles.

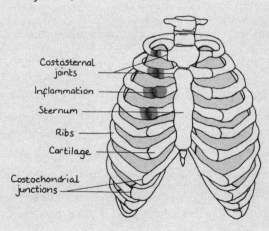

What causes breathlessness in Long Covid?

Let's look at the factors that may be contributing to symptoms of breathlessness in Long Covid, particularly when conventional investigations fail to identify a cause.

Some of the components that contribute to breathlessness are internal and some are external, which you may find more difficult to assess or control.

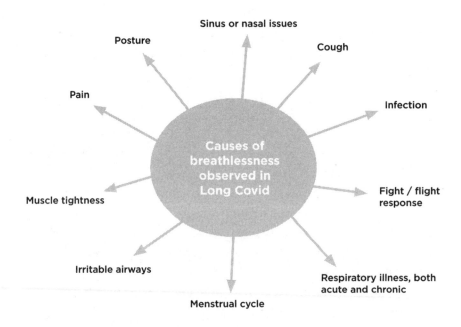

Let's explore how some of these can result in breathlessness.

Pain

Chest pains can be a feature of acute respiratory infections, such as pneumonia and Covid-19. The pain itself can alter how a person breathes. For example, a woman we assessed in clinic had pneumonia at the bottom of her left lung, which caused lung pain on deep breathing. As a result, she had modified her breathing to become shallow to avoid triggering the pain. To compensate for this less efficient way of breathing, she also started to breathe faster. This new breathing pattern then become habitual and months after the infection, even simple activities around the house made her breathless. You may also experience chest pain due to other causes (*see* chapter 8, Other Long Covid symptoms), including poor posture, coughing, and areas of inflammation. It is important to address these if possible as all of these can impact on your breathing pattern.

Anxiety

Why am I still unwell? What is wrong with my body? It's now been four weeks since I caught Covid and I still feel unwell. We know that anxiety induces adrenaline release and speeds up our heart and breathing rates. When this occurs against the background of already feeling breathless, it can result in higher levels of anxiety, which then fuels this cycle.

Muscle tightness/posture

Your posture can have a direct impact on your breathing. If you spend a great deal of time sitting down, this can restrict the movement of your diaphragm and cause increasing tension in your neck and shoulders. We often see overactive accessory muscles in the neck and upper chest affecting breathing. Abdominal muscles that are tight and contracted can also restrict expansion of the diaphragm.

FIGHT/FLIGHT RESPONSE

SARS-CoV2, the virus that causes Covid-19, primarily infects the lungs and upper airways. During the initial phase of the infection, your body releases stress hormones (such as adrenaline) that increase your breathing and heart rate to help tackle the infection. This is a completely normal physiological response to illness, and as you recover from the infection your breathing should return to normal. However, it is observed that in some people this does not happen and switching off the fight or flight (stress response) mode can be more of a challenge. This response is driven by the autonomic nervous system, part of the nervous system that regulates the automatic processes within your body, including heart rate, digestion, blood pressure and breathing. These are controlled by opposing systems: the sympathetic nervous system (SNS), which generates fight and flight responses (increasing blood pressure, breathing and heart rate), and the parasympathetic nervous system (PNS) that slows down these responses and is activated when our body is in a state of relaxation.

SNS – fight or flight mode, where we **expend** our energy.

PNS – rest, restore and digest mode, where we **conserve** our energy.

Many people with Long Covid describe feeling as though they are stuck in fight/flight mode, always feeling on edge or high alert. This directly affects the way in which you breathe. However, helpfully, controlling the way you breathe has a direct impact on stimulating the parasympathetic nervous system. By doing this, you turn on the restorative processes within your body that are essential for recovery.

'It felt as if I had been a train speeding along the track and had now been derailed and was stuck in a deep muddy field. I know now it was a vicious circle of stress and anxiety and I had developed an incorrect breathing pattern. I was stuck in a fight or flight mode. I was frightened and didn't understand why I wasn't getting better.'

How can you assess your own breathing pattern?

When you have identified the possible factors that may be contributing to your breathlessness following Covid-19, the next step is to analyse your breathing pattern. It is important to observe your own breathing so that as you learn the principles of how to breathe correctly, you can reassess to see if you are making progress.

Find somewhere quiet where you can be comfortable and have the opportunity to concentrate on your breathing. Ideally, this exercise is best performed lying with your head and neck comfortable on a pillow and your knees bent and supported either with a pillow or feet flat on the floor, with your hands resting on either your chest, tummy or sides of your ribs.

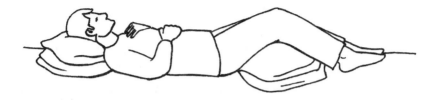

Then slowly work through the following steps:

- Notice any tension in your face, jaw, neck, shoulders, chest or stomach.
- Shift your awareness to any soreness, aches or pains.
- Listen to and feel your breathing – can you hear yourself breathing in or out?
- Notice if you are breathing through your nose or mouth or a combination of both.
- Do you breathe into your upper chest or down into your stomach?
- Is your breathing smooth or jumpy, deep or shallow?
- Do you want to take deep breaths, yawn or sigh, cough or clear your throat?
- Do you hold your breath?
- Do you feel that you need to think about your breathing?
- Time your breathing rate over 30 seconds.

'I was asked to take a deep breath, I just couldn't do it. When I breathed in, the inhalation came in judders and starts and my body felt wired, like it was on red alert. It was clear I had a breathing pattern disorder and I felt fearful of my breath.'

What is good breathing?

When you are looking to ensure you are breathing efficiently, it is important to understand what a good breathing pattern looks like. Physiotherapists often use the term Nose, Low, and Slow™. This was coined by BradCliff

Breathing physiotherapists and is designed specifically for their system of breathing retraining.

These terms can be helpful to remind you what makes a breathing pattern effective. Let's break them down.

Nose

Physiologically, you are designed to breathe in through the nose for a number of reasons. First, it warms and filters the air. Second, it allows you to slow down and control the rate and depth of your breath, ensuring that you utilise the diaphragm (the main muscle of breathing), and third, nasal breathing produces a gas called nitric oxide that promotes efficient gas exchange within the lungs. We often say to patients to remember that the **'nose is for breathing, mouth for eating'**!

If nasal breathing is difficult due to sinus issues, you may be able to use a nasal spray or perform nasal rinsing on a daily basis. These techniques assist in keeping the airways clear. There are specific products available for this that do not require a prescription. On occasions, a steroid-based nasal spray may be worth trying to settle any inflammation present. This is something you can discuss with your healthcare provider.

Low

The depth and direction of your breath in is important. By concentrating on utilising the lower part of your chest and your tummy, you ensure that the diaphragm muscle at the base of your lungs contracts down-wards and enables your lungs to fill with air, maximising absorption of oxygen. Over time, if breathing is performed using the top of the lungs (you may say it feels shallow), then the essential muscle of breathing – the diaphragm – will be underutilised and your breathing will become inefficient. After a while you may start to think, incorrectly, that upper chest breathing is required to create a satisfying breath. To correct this breathing pattern, you may need to consciously engage in abdominal breathing. This may feel odd at first, as does trying to break any habit, but with time and practice it will start to feel normal and automatic again.

The size of the breath you take is equally important. Healthy lungs have a capacity to contain around 4–6 litres of air, depending on your age, gender and ethnicity. When we breathe at rest, the volume of air that we move in and out (known as the tidal volume) is around 500ml. We can think about this as slightly bigger than a Coke can. People are often surprised by this as they believe that a bigger breath often means a better breath.

Slow

A normal breathing rate when you are fit and well is around 8 to 12 breaths per minute and this is optimal for your body to work efficiently. However, if your breathing is less efficient, this rate may not meet the demands of your body and to compensate for this, you have to breathe more often. By concentrating on the timing of the **in** and the **out** breath, you can start to regulate the rate at which you breathe. When first practising this, we would always recommend that the breath in to breath out timing is comfortable. We normally advise to start with a 2:3 timing. This means that you breathe in for the count of 2 and out for 3. If you find this hard to do, the most important aspect to concentrate on in the beginning is just focusing on breathing out more than in.

Some specialist breathing practices in holistic therapies such as yoga, Pilates or mindfulness advocate much longer inspiration to expiration times, which can be very beneficial. However, is it important when retraining your breathing, and dedicating time to correcting a breathing pattern, that you keep it simple and comfortable.

Good breathing practice

Now that we have looked at the most important aspects of breathing, the key thing is to practise and continually reassess. We recommend that the best position to practise good breathing is on your back in the same conditions that we asked you to assess your breathing (comfortable, warm and relaxed).

- Lie on your back with your head, neck and shoulders completely relaxed into a pillow or cushion and a pillow under your knees. Place your feet in the 10 and 2 o'clock position. The aim is to switch off those postural, abdominal and accessory breathing muscles as much as possible (*see* image p. 61)
- Place your hands on your tummy just below the tummy button, with your fingertips touching and your elbows relaxed down by your side.

- Concentrating on the tips discussed above, notice how the breath in moves quietly through the nose, down low into the tummy, and is slow and controlled.
- The breath out is a passive movement and should not be forced. It should feel like a relaxation of the muscles.

AIR HUNGER

As you begin to practise, you may experience the sensation of air hunger, or an urge to take a deep breath. This is completely normal as your body may be stuck in a habitual pattern and is therefore uncomfortable with what you are now asking it to do. Ideally you want to try to work through this for as long as you can. You can do this by attempting to swallow the urge away, counting a further 3–4 breaths and then taking a deep breath or using other forms of distraction, for example music or visual aids (as discussed later in the chapter). As you continue to dedicate time to practising good breathing, these urges should lessen, until you are able to complete a 10-minute session with no urges at all.

'I found it REALLY hard over the first 48 hours to resist the urge to gasp for breath / take the deep breath that my body seemed to crave. So, I kept monitoring my sats to reassure myself that my body was getting adequate oxygen regardless. And now, I have been able to control my breathing much more naturally and these days, when I find myself lapsing into old habits again, I find myself catching it early and becoming more mindful and finding it easier to quickly reset the breath.'

How often should I practise?

In order to retrain the brain, tap into the correct neural pathways, and encourage correct activation of the primary muscles for breathing, we suggest that these exercises are practised on a regular basis throughout the day. In our clinic, we recommend three separate 10-minute sessions spread across the day. Many people report that doing 10 minutes before going to bed really helps to calm down the body and prepare them for sleep. It is important to plan these sessions into your day to make them part of your normal routine. If you are also experiencing fatigue, these breathing exercises can be incorporated into your restorative and restful breaks in your day. Equally, they can be used to calm down the fight/flight response in the body during times of rising anxiety or stressful situations.

'I find the exercises are especially beneficial to calm down my panic and regulate my breathing with longer breaths and I feel my muscles relax.'

'I learnt that this way of breathing was stimulating the "rest digest" parasympathetic part of the autonomic nervous system, rather than the fight/flight sympathetic. I now do this "breathing retraining" twice a day for 10–15 minutes and I check in with myself several times a day that my breath is slow. If I don't practise this every day, I feel the juddery breathing pattern and other symptoms returning.'

TIPS AND TRICKS FOR PRACTISING BREATHING CONTROL

- Look for a rectangle shape in the room, e.g. a window, door or TV screen. Move around the sides of the rectangle with your eyes, breathing in on the short sides and out on the long sides. This can help to lengthen the expiration breath.

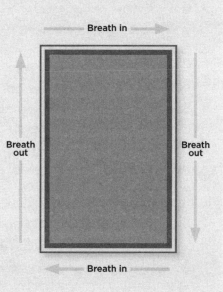

- Using a wide straw (this is important as it should not be difficult or increase the resistance to breathing out), blow bubbles into a glass of water as you slowly breathe out. Ensure the breath in continues via the nose. This also helps to extend the expiration phase of the breathing cycle.

  'It gave me a lot of joy blowing bubbles through a straw! Takes me back to blowing bubbles into strawberry milkshake as a child!'

- When lying down practising breathing control, you may find it useful to adopt the BradCliff beach pose™ with your hands above your head. This helps to 'switch off' those accessory muscles and reduce the amount of movement in your upper chest when you are attempting to control your breathing.
- Place a standard-sized hardback book on your stomach when practising tummy breathing to aid awareness of the depth of breath. People often say watching the rise and fall of the book can help as a visual stimulus.
- Use your family or work colleagues around you to help observe your breathing and notice if it starts to become shallower and faster. They can be great reassurers if you educate them on why you may breathe abnormally, and help you to feel safe, reiterating how to regain control.
- Using a hand-held fan directed towards the face can reduce the sensation of breathlessness; placing a cool flannel on the face can do the same.
- Relaxation – it is important to practise these exercises when your body feels in a relaxed state. It can be useful to do a short mindfulness exercise or meditation session beforehand if you are familiar with these. Alternatively, take a moment to do a 'body scan' and notice where you may have tightness and/ or discomfort, focusing on relaxing these muscles or areas of tension.

'I rely on breathing exercises when my symptoms return as a way of gaining control.'

'It really has made a difference to my quality of life in the past few days. Such a small thing, such a big impact.'

How can I progress this into activity?

As you become more comfortable with the breathing technique in the lying position, you can start to progress into sitting, then standing, before eventually progressing into walking and stair climbing. As your level of exertion increases, it is natural for your breathing and heart rate to rise and for you to start breathing through your mouth. However, when you are walking on the flat at your own pace, aim to keep your breathing quiet and continue to breathe through the nose as much as you can. This may be particularly difficult at the start but will get easier with practice.

TIPS TO TRY WHEN WALKING, CLIMBING STAIRS AND INCREASING GENERAL ACTIVITY

- If you find it more difficult to breathe through your nose, you can try breathing out through pursed lips. You can imagine this as gently blowing on a candle to make it flicker.

- If you feel breathless when exerting yourself, or at any time, one saying that many therapists use is to **stop, drop and flop**! BradCliff: Stop Drop Flop™

  - **Stop** what you are doing and check your breathing pattern.

  - **Drop**, resting a hand on your tummy and taking low, slow abdominal breaths in and out through the nose.

  - **Flop**, relax your neck muscles and shoulder girdle, breathing out through your mouth.

- Before reaching forwards or bending over to pick something up, take a slow and low breath in through your nose, and then breathe out as you come back up. The term **'blow as you go'** is often used to help people remember to breathe out during the effort part of an activity.

- When climbing the stairs or an incline or walking at a faster pace, it can be useful to pace your breathing with your steps. An example of this may be breathing in for 2 steps and then out for 3, or in for 3 and out for 4. It is important to find the most comfortable and natural counting sequence for you and this is likely to change over time as you become more relaxed with the breathing techniques.

- Always check in with your breathing at regular intervals and make sure you are not holding your breath or breathing in too much and over-inflating or 'hyper-inflating' your lungs – **'if in doubt, breathe out!'** BradCliff™

- It can be very useful to practise breathing control before and after activity to reduce the sensations of breathlessness and allow you to feel more in control.

Useful positions to aid breathlessness

When you become breathless, it isn't always appropriate to lie down on the floor and practise the exercises we have described. The diagrams opposite show a number of positions that people find useful to help them regain control of their breathing, utilising the BradCliff Nose, Low and Slow™ technique.

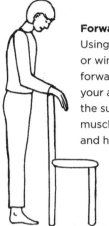

Forward lean standing

Using a chair, table or windowsill, lean forwards and rest your arms gently on the surface. Keep the muscles in your arms and hands relaxed.

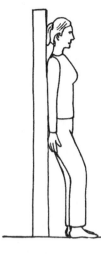

Standing with wall support

Facing away from a wall, place your feet slightly apart and approximately 30cm (12in) in front of you, and lean back against the wall for support. Rest your arms by your sides.

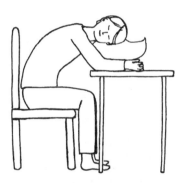

Forward lean sitting – with table

Lean forward from the waist over a table, and rest your head and neck on one or two pillows. Your arms can be resting over the top of the pillow or on the table.

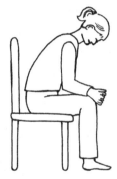

Forward lean sitting – without table

Lean forward from the waist and rest your elbows on your thighs. Keep the muscles in your arms and hands relaxed.

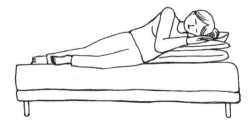

High side lying

Lying on either side with your knees slightly bent, prop your upper body up on pillows, ensuring your head and neck are supported.

TIPS FOR BREATHING AND TALKING ADAPTED FROM BRADCLIFF™

The voice is produced by the flow of air striking the vocal folds as you breathe out. The throat, tongue, lips and soft palate then modify the sound. The diaphragm controls the breath and so any alteration in the way in which you breathe can contribute to voice issues or increased breathlessness when you are talking.

- Breathe slowly through your nose between sentences while talking, instead of quickly gasping air into the upper chest through the mouth.
- Progress to taking small sips of air in through your mouth between sentences, ensuring the air moves low and slow into the tummy.
- Put mental commas into your speech to create pauses.
- Practise speaking in front of a mirror – for example, recite the alphabet slowly. Start very slowly and purposefully. Sit down, relax the neck/shoulder girdle/upper chest, breathe in through your nose and into your tummy, then say, 'A' slowly, using all the air you just breathed in to make the sound. Pause for a moment, and then repeat, saying, 'B' and so on.
- Practise reading aloud from a book and record yourself. Monitor your progress by repeating this every couple of weeks.
- Listen to your own answerphone message so you can observe if you're speaking fast and sound breathless when talking.
- Watch other people's breathing habits when they speak and listen during telephone conversations.
- Continue to focus on the Nose, Low and Slow™ techniques learnt.

'The tip of putting a mental comma into a sentence, slowing down my pattern of speech, taking a small nasal breath between sentences and considering what I wanted or needed to say, made speaking on the phone or on a Zoom call easier, less tiring and more mindful.'

TIPS FOR BREATHING AND EATING

- Avoid eating on the run: sit down to eat and avoid talking with your mouth full. This can often lead to air gulping and bloating. Eat very small mouthfuls if you are experiencing sensations of tightness in the throat.
- Think about your posture when you are eating, as being slumped in a low chair can cause the stomach to restrict diaphragm movement.
- Drink small sips to prevent air gulping. Drinking through a straw is a good way to practise sipping and swallowing, in conjunction with breathing to avoid swallowing air.

COUGHING

A common symptom seen during the acute phase of Covid is a dry cough. We also see this as a continuing symptom in Long Covid.

Coughing is a natural bodily response that assists in clearing the airways and throat of material. This may be a foreign body (e.g. food) or sputum (mucus or phlegm). However, a cough may also be a symptom of an underlying condition. If it persists for more than eight weeks, it is advisable that you see your healthcare provider in the first instance. If no cause is found, then it is likely that the cough serves no useful purpose and has become habitual. Frequent coughing increases energy expenditure and over time can become exhausting. It can also cause chest or rib pain and irritate the airways and larynx (voice box), increasing the need to cough and triggering a vicious cycle.

If an underlying cause for the cough has been excluded, it is worth taking steps to control it to reduce the impact it is having on your life. Here are some general tips and tricks that you may find helpful. As with other Long Covid self-management strategies, the more you practise, the easier it becomes to incorporate these approaches into your daily routine.

- Using the breathing control techniques advised, particularly nasal breathing, can help to reduce the irritation caused in the throat and upper airways.
- Ensure you are drinking plenty throughout the day and have water handy at night. This can help to keep the throat hydrated and reduce tickly sensations that may be present.
- Avoid or reduce use of caffeinated drinks, as these can increase your cough.
- Avoid external irritants such as smoke or perfumes, which can irritate the airways and encourage coughing and heartburn.
- If you have the sensation of needing to cough, you can try 'swallowing the cough away' or sucking on a boiled sweet or ice cubes to ease the throat.
- If you use regular inhalers, ensure you have your technique checked regularly as a poor technique can stimulate a cough. If using a steroid inhaler, ensure you are rinsing your mouth after using it to reduce residue in the throat, which can be aggravating.

FURTHER SUPPORT

If you continue to experience symptoms associated with breathlessness, we would advise that you seek further evaluation from your healthcare provider and support from a qualified physiotherapist, who can complete a full assessment and provide an individualised approach to breathing retraining.

SUMMARY

- Breathlessness is one of the most common symptoms in Long Covid and can be frightening and disabling.

- For most people with Long Covid, standard investigations for breathlessness are usually normal, and do not show evidence of lung damage.

- In the Long Covid clinic, we see many people struggling with breathlessness. Changes in the way you breathe can contribute to this, and may result in many of the other symptoms discussed in this chapter. This is known as Breathing Pattern Disorder.

- By practising the strategies and techniques we have explained, you can learn to take control of your breathing, reset your breathing pattern, and reduce the sensation of breathlessness.

CHAPTER 4

Sleep and Long Covid

In this chapter, we explain the basics of normal sleep, outline the common problems that contribute to poor sleep in people with Long Covid and provide tips on how to improve sleep quality. We also look at the most common sleep disorder, obstructive sleep apnoea (OSA), which may merit consideration in people who are excessively sleepy.

The impact of poor sleep

We are still in the process of understanding how the SARS-CoV-2 virus causes the range of symptoms we see in Long Covid. Some symptoms are straightforward to explain, such as loss of smell (due to damage of the olfactory nerve pathways), but other symptoms, such as fatigue and disrupted sleep, are less clear cut. Poor sleep is a feature of many health conditions and can have a major influence on how unwell we feel, and almost always affects how we cope with our symptom burden.

Many people struggling with Long Covid describe disruption to their normal sleeping pattern, which may compromise sleep quality. The impact of poor sleep is wide reaching, affecting cognitive functions such as memory, processing and reasoning. It also affects our emotional and psychological health and, in the longer term, increases the risk of serious medical and psychological problems. Many people with Long Covid find that poor sleep worsens almost all other symptoms, but particularly fatigue and brain fog. Conversely, following a restful night's sleep, these symptoms are often eased and people report feeling better able to manage the day ahead.

'I've got two kids and I know what sleep deprivation feels like.
This was the next level. I was SO tired but if I was lucky enough to

fall asleep I would wake up within minutes as if I had been injected with a litre of coffee. Exhausting.'

The ways in which Long Covid impacts on sleep vary between individuals. You may find it difficult getting off to sleep or you may fall asleep easily but have problems staying asleep, waking early in the morning or at intervals through the night. For some, vivid or unpleasant dreams can be a problem. For others, sleeping for too long can be as much of an issue as not getting enough good-quality sleep.

Most people with Long Covid report that they no longer feel refreshed by sleep. In the Long Covid clinic, if sleep is a problem, we often ask about sleeping habits, including the time you go to sleep and the time you wake up in the morning. Looking at the reasons you wake at night (if known) can be useful to help us to understand the factors contributing to poor sleep. These questions may also identify people who have a sleep disorder, such as obstructive sleep apnoea, that may have developed or become worse after having Covid.

Sleep

Sleep is vitally important to our health and well-being. It is as fundamental as eating or drinking. We spend roughly one-third of each day asleep and this time is key to forming memories, learning, processing emotions and good physical health.

Sleep pressure

There are two processes that control sleep (see figure 1). The first is something we refer to as 'sleep pressure'. This is the growing need (or pressure) for sleep that builds up during the day as the number of hours we are awake lengthens. Some circumstances can increase sleep pressure, such as illness (including infection), mentally challenging activities and increased physical activity.

Body clock

The second process is our body clock (also called the circadian rhythm), which is controlled by daylight hours Daylight in the morning helps us to wake up and darkness in the evening makes us sleepy. This is because darkness stimulates the brain to produce a hormone called melatonin, which is crucial in controlling our body clock. Rising melatonin levels and increased sleep pressure (due to the hours we have been awake) work in combination to help us get a good night's sleep. Therefore, activities that interrupt either of these can make it harder for us to get to sleep. For example, exposure to light late in the evening (particularly the blue light emitted by electronic screens) can delay the release of melatonin, while napping in the daytime reduces sleep pressure and the drive to fall asleep at night.

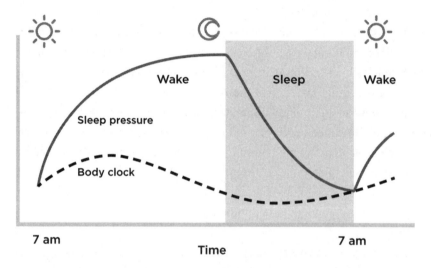

FIGURE 1: The two processes that control sleep are sleep pressure and the body clock or circadian rhythm. After waking, sleep pressure builds up throughout the day, increasing the need for sleep. In the morning, daylight wakes up our body clock, keeping us alert until sunset. Dusk triggers melatonin release, which, together with increasing sleep pressure, makes us sleepy. At night, sleeping resets our sleep pressure, allowing us to wake up refreshed in the morning.

HOW MUCH SLEEP DO WE NEED?

People need different amounts of sleep to function normally. Most people sleep between seven and nine hours per night. However, you may be one of those people who normally manage well with less than seven hours (lucky you!) or be on the sleepier end of the scale and need more than nine hours of sleep each night.

Modern lifestyles, with busy schedules and electronic screens, often disturb the normal processes controlling sleep and prevent people getting enough sleep. Reducing sleep duration to less than six hours long term has been linked with an increased risk of health problems, including diabetes, high blood pressure and heart disease.

Good-quality sleep

The quality of sleep is also important. To achieve this, your brain needs to be able to cycle through the different phases of sleep naturally (see the Sleep Cycle box below).

Sleep cycles can vary from person to person and from night to night based on a wide range of factors (age, alcohol consumption, medications). Each cycle lasts approximately 90 minutes and we generally have between four and six cycles per night. The first cycle is often the shortest, while later cycles tend to be a bit longer. It is common to come closer to the surface of waking or even waking up at the end of the cycle before drifting off into the next. Some people complain that they often wake at the same time each night; however, this is just a sign that the internal body clock is working well and with regularity.

Surprisingly, sleeping excessively is also associated with physical and psychological problems, and may over time contribute to loss of physical fitness and fatigue, alongside other problems such as headache, low mood and pain.

THE SLEEP CYCLE

When we initially fall asleep, our muscles relax and our breathing and heart rate slow. After this, we cycle through lighter phases of sleep (termed stages 1 and 2); we then move into deeper sleep, referred to as stage 3, and REM (rapid eye movement) sleep. During REM sleep, there is almost complete paralysis of the muscles, apart from the breathing muscles and eye muscles. Your eyes move quickly under your eyelids during this sleep stage (hence the name) and this is when most dreaming occurs. These deeper stages of sleep are believed to benefit learning, memory and mood. Therefore, a reduction in these stages may impair memory formation, learning and emotional processing. Over time, this can physiologically stress the body and increase the risk of medical problems. Irregular sleep patterns, broken sleep and sleep disorders reduce this restorative deep sleep. Medications (including sleeping tablets) and alcohol may make it feel easier for you to get to sleep but impair the ability of your brain to reach the deeper depths of sleep and so have a negative effect on your sleep quality overall.

Sleep in Long Covid

When we are unwell with an infection, including Covid, we generally need to sleep and rest more. This is an important physiological response as it improves the ability of our immune system to fight infection. The restorative process of sleep is also essential during the recovery period and assists with healing. Indeed, after we have been acutely unwell, we often feel washed out and exhausted for some weeks as our body recovers. People who have been critically unwell with Covid often find that they need to sleep for a few hours more each night, and may also find that they need additional sleep in the day. This is completely normal, and after weeks or months, the hours of sleep required usually start to reduce back down towards normal.

In many people with Long Covid, however, sleep problems are not related to too much sleeping, but rather with poor-quality sleep. People often lose their normal sleep pattern, or find their sleep is interrupted and fragmented. Many struggle to fall asleep at night. While there are many factors that contribute to poor sleep quality in Long Covid, there are some more common contributing causes. As you read through the following paragraphs, have a think about which of these may be playing a role in your sleep issues, and then consider whether the following guidance may help you get a better night's sleep.

Fatigue

As we saw in chapter 2, fatigue and tiredness are not the same. Tiredness is a normal part of life and signals the need for sleep. Usually, after a good night's sleep, energy levels are restored and the feeling of tiredness resolves. Fatigue is more persistent and pervasive than this, with the feeling of whole-body tiredness, more often described as exhaustion, that can limit normal functioning and is only partially (or temporarily) relieved by sleep. People sometimes describe feeling completely empty of energy or washed out.

However, although there are differences, the two are intricately linked. When we are tired, we also feel fatigued; when we are fatigued, we generally feel tired. So to help improve fatigue levels, good-quality sleep is essential.

It is instinctive that when we feel tired or fatigued, we seek rest. Napping during the day can sometimes be helpful and enable us to get through to bedtime and undertake essential daily tasks such as cooking dinner and looking after children. Prolonged naps can be counterproductive, however. After around 20 minutes, we start to enter the deeper phases of sleep and while these then reduce the sleep pressure, they will offset the sleep-wake rhythm of the brain and make it difficult to get to sleep at night or to stay asleep through the night. People who nap during the day often describe a restless, light sleep at night, with frequent awakenings. The temptation then is to stay in bed and try to sleep in to compensate for the poor night's sleep. This then further offsets the body clock and disturbs the sleep pattern, ultimately perpetuating the feeling of tiredness and fatigue. Good sleep hygiene can help (*see* p.82).

Loss of normal routine

Long Covid can have a big impact on working lives and many people with the condition are unable to return to their normal daily schedules. This loss of usual routine may result in relaxing or changing your usual bedtime routine, and the times you go to bed and get up may vary day-to-day. This reduction in physical and mental activity may reduce sleep pressure and although you often feel tired, you may find you struggle to fall and stay asleep.

Reduced physical exercise

Most people we see with Long Covid were previously fit and well, and exercise was part of their daily or weekly routine. Moderate aerobic exercise has been shown to improve sleep quality, making it easier for people to fall asleep and reach deeper stages of restorative sleep.

Feeling fatigued and unwell with Long Covid does not make exercise easy or appealing. Some people struggle with simple daily activities, such as getting dressed and making breakfast, and so the amount of physical activity undertaken is hugely reduced. It is also common in Long Covid to experience worsening fatigue following exercise and on occasions it can leave people wiped out for several days afterwards.

Unfortunately, there is not a 'quick fix' for this problem and it is essential to build up levels of physical activity slowly and at your own pace. While you may not be able to engage in your previous level of physical activity, there may be small elements that you could incorporate into your day. The amount you can do is individual to you and further advice regarding this can be found in chapter 5 (Return to Physical Activity).

Psychological health

Disrupted sleep is common in Long Covid and the consequences of poor-quality sleep increase the chances that you will experience mood disturbance, anxiety and depression. For some people, having chronic Long Covid symptoms, and the frustration of being unwell, causes a great deal of stress and worry, which can impact directly on sleep quality. It may also be that anxiety and low mood existed to an extent prior to getting Covid but that these problems have been made much worse since becoming unwell.

Anxiety and chronic stress are associated with increased physiological arousal in which hormones (cortisol and adrenaline) are released in the body and create the 'fight or flight' or sympathetic response. While this has advantages in moments of emergency or high pressure, it is not helpful for getting to sleep. People who suffer with anxiety often struggle to get off to sleep, wake frequently in the night or in the early hours of the morning and are unable to get back to sleep. Others feel a sense of having slept very lightly and of waking at the smallest thing. Good-quality sleep switches off the 'fight or flight' sympathetic response and activates the parasympathetic nervous system, which slows down your heart rate and breathing and induces a state of relaxation. Doing a relaxing activity or listening to a guided relaxation before bed might help with getting off to sleep if you think anxiety and stress interferes with your sleep at night.

Disrupted, poor-quality sleep is a risk factor for depression and, similarly, sleep problems frequently coexist in people with depression. Early-morning wakening is a common feature of depression and, less commonly, excessive sleepiness can also be a sign. If you struggle with low mood or chronic anxiety, it could be worthwhile discussing this further with your healthcare practitioner.

When you are unwell, it is common to worry about the consequences of poor sleep, but putting pressure on yourself to get a really good night's sleep can be counterproductive and lead to a vicious cycle of poor sleep. This can be tricky to get out of and cognitive behavioural therapy (CBT), a talking therapy that helps you manage your thoughts or behaviour, can be useful for these sorts of problems. CBT-i (CBT-insomnia) is CBT specifically designed for people with insomnia and can be particularly helpful.

NIGHTMARES/VIVID DREAMS/PTSD

It is not unusual to experience bad dreams after a traumatic experience such as having been ill with Covid, as dreams often reflect what has happened during our daily life. Many people suffering with Long Covid report vivid or bad dreams; some also describe flashbacks to events related to their acute illness, although, for others, the content is not representative of their experiences.

'All things considered, I feel like one of the lucky ones and I am pleased with how I have done since leaving hospital. My mood is quite up and down though, and I sometimes get flashbacks to being in intensive care. I have a dream where I am looking down on myself from above, when I'm on a ventilator, as they are about to turn me onto my front.'

For some people, the fear associated with their acute illness (especially if night-time breathlessness was experienced) never completely eases and sufferers may still feel afraid to go to sleep. This may be more apparent in patients who were treated in hospital and required oxygen via a mask or admission to intensive care.

Flashbacks and vivid dreams or nightmares are not uncommon after these experiences and may be a sign of post-traumatic stress disorder (PTSD). If you are struggling with these symptoms, it would be worth discussing them with your healthcare practitioner.

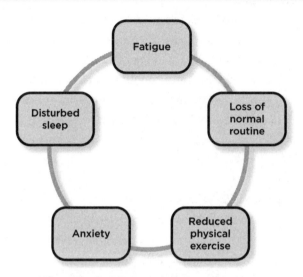

FIGURE 2: Factors leading to disturbed sleep in Long Covid. Fatigue is a very common symptom in people with Long Covid. Fatigue often leads to a loss of normal routine and reduced physical exercise. These factors, coupled with anxiety – which is often exacerbated by Long Covid and the ongoing Covid-19 pandemic – can lead to disturbed sleep, which in itself will likely worsen fatigue.

Practical management

Having looked at several reasons sleep problems develop after Covid-19, you can see how interconnected these problems are. So, let's look at some ways to help improve sleep, regardless of contributing factors.

Sleep hygiene

Adopting a healthy sleeping routine and avoiding behaviour that negatively impacts on the quality of sleep is essential. A set of measures to help improve sleep quality is called **sleep hygiene**. Although some of the advice might seem a bit obvious, it is often not followed by many of us who are struggling with sleep problems. As you read through the advice, think about whether you have been following the principles, and if not, try adopting them to see how this impacts your sleep quality over the next few weeks.

Sleep schedule

- Keep a regular bedtime and anchor your wake-up time. This helps with your body clock and supports your sleep.
- Keep your bedtime routine at approximately the same time on working and non-working days.
- Aim to wake up at around the same time at the weekends. Try to avoid 'catching up' on missed sleep or sleeping in too much at the weekends, as getting up later makes it harder to feel sleepy at bedtime.
- If you are a shift worker, try to minimise night-to-night variation in bedtime for the majority of nights.

During the day

- Morning daylight has been proved to be essential in maintaining a good body clock and thus helping you to get a better night's sleep. If you can, go outside in natural daylight for at least 10 minutes in the morning, even if this is just in your garden or close to home.
- Depending on the stage you are at in your recovery, regular physical activity can help build some 'sleep pressure' to feel tired in the evening

DAYTIME NAPS

- If you are at the stage with your energy levels where you need to nap during the day, plan these as part of your daily schedule (see chapter 2 on Managing Fatigue).
- Try not to nap from mid to late afternoon onwards as this can be too close to your bedtime and reduces sleep pressure.
- Keep naps to a maximum of 20 minutes, setting an alarm before you rest or nap (otherwise, you enter into the deeper stages of sleep, which can interfere with your night-time sleep).
- Nap somewhere other than your bedroom, keeping your bedroom just for night-time sleep and intimacy.

(*see* chapter 2 on Managing Fatigue and chapter 5 on Return to Physical Activity).

- Physical activity at a low–moderate intensity may help with your sleep. Try to form a habit and, if possible, do this during the day rather than close to the time you go to sleep at night.
- Avoiding caffeine after midday can often help if you are struggling with sleep. Approximately 25 per cent of the caffeine in a cup of coffee remains in the body around 12 hours after drinking it.
- Limit your overall caffeine intake to a minimum and consider trying decaffeinated alternatives. Remember, caffeinated drinks include most energy drinks and fizzy drinks as well as tea and coffee.
- Avoid alcohol, particularly after 6 p.m. While alcohol may make you feel sleepy, it is known to worsen sleep quality and affect your mood.

Before bed:
- Make some time to relax and wind down in the evening. As part of this, you might want to use some time to reflect or talk through any of the day's events or plan activities for the next day, rather than doing this close to bedtime.
- There are lots of techniques for relaxing and de-stressing before bedtime to help you fall asleep more quickly, including relaxing music, breathing exercises and meditation. There are guided relaxations available to help with this that can be downloaded as apps or found on the internet.
- Having a warm bath or shower 1–2 hours before bed is relaxing, and facilitates the natural cooling of your body temperature afterwards, which helps prepare you for sleep.
- Have a pen/pencil and paper to hand by your bed. If you find yourself running over things in your mind, write your thoughts down, safe in the knowledge that they will be there for you to deal with at a more convenient moment.

Bedroom environment
- Try to keep your bedroom for sleep and intimacy only.
- If possible, find another environment in which to work or relax; this helps give your brain the message that your bedroom is for sleep.

- If this is not possible, create different 'zones' in your room to complete these other tasks, keeping your bed for sleep.
- Ensure that your bedroom is as comfortable as you can possibly make it: cool but not too cold, dark and quiet.
  — Blackout curtains or blinds can help.
  — Earplugs can be useful.
- Keep electronic devices like phones, tablets, laptops and TVs out of the bedroom.
- Consider switching off half the lights at home a few hours before bed. Better still, switch to candlelight – this emits a spectrum of light that does not have the negative effects of light emitted from devices in the evening.
- Avoid using your phone as an alarm clock to avoid the distraction of keeping your phone in the bedroom.
- Keep pets out of the bedroom, particularly if they are noisy or restless and decide they want to wake you at night.

Electronic screens, such as laptops, computers, tablets and smartphones, all contain a blue light that suppresses the release of melatonin (the sleepy hormone). In the day, blue light (which is also emitted from the sun) can be helpful as it enables us to feel more alert. However, too close to bedtime and it can trick the body into thinking it is still daytime. Some people say they don't think that using devices at bedtime stops them from getting to sleep – but it could be interfering with the *quality* of your sleep. That, coupled with the often more stimulating and engaging activity people do on such devices, can disrupt a good night's sleep. Although night screen modes reduce the amount of blue light emitted by electronic screens, avoiding using devices for at least an hour prior to bed is advisable.

'I knew that I had fallen into poor sleep habits so I started setting an alarm when I napped so I wouldn't sleep for so long. I would need to do this at least a couple of times a day and was terrified about returning to work due to how tired I felt. My line manager was really understanding though and would let me go to my car for

a short nap in the afternoon, which really helped. Although I am still exhausted by the end of the day, I am now sleeping pretty solidly through the night and no longer need a sleep in the day. A good night's sleep makes it possible for me to see the light at the end of the tunnel, but I am still a far way off feeling back to normal.'

Obstructive sleep apnoea

Obstructive sleep apnoea (OSA) is a medical condition affecting breathing during sleep. The muscles of the upper airway (throat) relax during sleep, and narrowing of the upper airway leads to vibration and snoring and, if the airway closes further, to pauses in breathing. These often terminate with a loud snore, or coughing and choking, and may be associated with a lightening of sleep or waking up. The result may be daytime tiredness, sleepiness, and impaired memory and concentration. Sleepiness is different to tiredness, in that sleepiness refers to difficulty in staying awake and an urge to fall asleep.

Some people visit their doctor thinking they have insomnia, when in fact OSA is causing them to wake at night and they are unable to get back to sleep. Risk factors for OSA are older age, male gender, being overweight, large tonsils and a backwards-set lower jaw, though it affects many other people too. If you are sleepy in the daytime and if you snore loudly, or if anyone has ever noticed pauses in your breathing during your sleep, you should discuss with your healthcare provider whether you may have OSA, as this could be contributing to your tiredness and fatigue (in addition to other Long Covid symptoms). You may be asked to fill in a questionnaire that can help to show whether you are at risk of obstructive sleep apnoea. A sleep study may be arranged, which is usually performed in your home and involves wearing equipment that records your oxygen levels, heart rate and other measures such as airflow, sound, markers of sleep disruption and chest movements.

Treatments for obstructive sleep apnoea depend on how people are affected. Those with mild or no daytime symptoms can manage OSA with weight loss, reducing alcohol and stopping sedating medications. However, those with marked symptoms may need treatment with continuous positive airway pressure (CPAP). CPAP is a snug-fitting face mask attached to a bedside machine that gently blows air on to the back of the throat to help open up the upper airway and stop snoring and pauses in breathing (this is the same type of treatment given to people in hospital with severe Covid infection who need support with their breathing). Another treatment for OSA is a jaw advancement device, a specialised mouth guard, often fitted by dentists, to be worn over your teeth while you sleep. It works by bringing your bottom teeth and jaw forwards to reduce snoring and can also reduce OSA.

'I have always been a snorer, and my wife used to tell me that sometimes I stopped breathing in my sleep and she had to poke me to get me to start again. When I was recovering from Covid, my snoring was even worse and I felt tired in the daytime and would fall asleep watching TV and even sitting in the car while my wife was driving – going on a ten-minute drive to the supermarket would send me to sleep.

'I spoke to my doctor, who sent me for a sleep study, which showed I had sleep apnoea. I met with a specialist who recommended CPAP, a mask worn at night that helps me to breathe while I sleep. At first I struggled to get to sleep due to the feeling of the mask, but I kept going with it and now I couldn't do without it. I have much more energy in the daytime and no longer doze off so easily. My wife is also happy as she is getting a better night's sleep, too!'

SUMMARY

- Sleep problems are common in Long Covid but they can be improved by following some simple tips.

- Improving your sleep can help your energy levels, making it easier to cope with other symptoms and manage daily activities.

- Having a regular routine and adopting good sleep hygiene may not lead to a perfect night's sleep but is likely to make a difference to your sleep quality over time.

- Obstructive sleep apnoea (OSA) can cause excessive daytime sleepiness. If you snore heavily or have pauses in your breathing when you sleep, it may be worth discussing this further with your healthcare provider.

CHAPTER 5

Return to Physical Activity

In this chapter, we are going to take you through the advice and strategies that have helped patients we have met in the Long Covid clinic, and guide you, whatever your circumstances, to your return to physical activity. We hope that this advice will help you recognise where you are currently, set realistic goals, and become more active.

Where you are now

You are probably reading this book because you have been affected by symptoms of Long Covid and want to get back to your normal self, in part by returning to a level of physical activity that you were previously used to. Or perhaps, after having Covid, you may wish to be more physically active than you were before you were ill. You might also have some concerns about doing exercise.

We are learning more about Covid and understand that it may affect the body differently to many of the viruses we are familiar with. It is normal after any viral infection, or period of illness, for it to take a little time for our activity levels and fitness levels to fully return. For those who have had Covid, the process of recovery can sometimes be prolonged and take months (possibly years) rather than days or weeks.

Although tempting, it is important not to keep looking back to when you found it so much easier to be physically active. The starting point on your return to physical activity needs to be set at the stage you are at now, in the present. You can then look forward to progressing to the exercise activities you previously enjoyed.

Expectations

The symptoms of Covid can affect anyone, from those who rarely exercise to elite athletes aiming to reach the top. It can leave you feeling tired and

weak, short of breath and with muscle and chest pains even when performing simple day-to-day tasks. This can be demoralising and leave you feeling
down. It is important to remember that you are not alone.

We recognise that even if you had mild symptoms when you were diag-
nosed with Covid, this does not necessarily mean that you will have an easy
recovery. Your symptoms many months later might well feel worse than
during the initial illness. For example, a short walk with your dog may be
exhausting, while doing things at home like gardening, housework or even
walking upstairs may leave you feeling tired and frustrated. It is therefore
important to set realistic expectations, which might be quite different to the
ambitions and goals you had prior to becoming unwell. As you recover, you
will need to listen to your body to help you find the right balance between
rest and physical activity and recognise that this may take some time.

Before you get started

Since these might be the first steps on a road towards higher levels of physical activity, it is very worthwhile looking into your motivations. As for
anyone exercising, it is important to find something you enjoy doing. Use
this time to reflect upon the types of physical activity you could enjoy on
a consistent basis. Take some time to think – and even write about – your
answers to the following questions:

- How did physical activity fit into my life before becoming unwell
  with Covid?
- What activities have I really enjoyed in the past?
- How important is it to me to increase my activity level currently?
- How confident am I that I will be able to increase my activity levels?

Goal setting

The idea of becoming more active and making changes can sometimes feel
quite daunting.

Setting goals can help you keep focused and motivated. This could make
things more manageable, given how you might be feeling with your symptoms. It is great to consider short-term goals so that making changes feels
more achievable. When setting goals, it is useful to keep them **SMART**.

BE SMART

- **Specific.** The goal should make clear what you want to accomplish – for example, 'to walk up the hill near home without stopping'.
- **Measurable.** Identify a way to measure and track progress towards the goal – for example, 'to increase the number of lamp-posts I walk to each week or two'.
- **Attainable.** Choosing very hard goals may be too challenging to achieve, so make them easy and realistic. For example, if you are not currently active, rather than 'go for a run', a better goal would be to walk at a fast pace on a short route near home without stopping.
- **Relevant.** Make goals relevant to important things in your life. For instance, walking at a fast pace from home to visit family and friends who live on the route you choose to take, or to go out on your bike with your children.
- **Time-framed.** Think about how frequently and for how long you will do the activity. In the early stages of recovery, this may be just a few minutes at a time, spread throughout the day and interspersed with longer than usual rest periods.

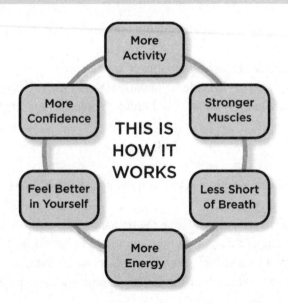

Physical activity and post-exertional malaise

Your symptoms, experience and life circumstances are unique. What activities you are able or unable to do are individual to you. This means that your focus may be different to other people with Long Covid. Your goals might be focused around your activities of daily living, such as domestic tasks and day-to-day errands, going back to work at full capacity, or returning to daily exercise. Your physical activity includes what you do in your free time, carrying out your usual daily tasks, and what you do when you are at work or school.

It is normal to feel tired after physical exertion but then to recover quickly after a rest or a good night's sleep. When fatigue worsens 12 to 48 hours after activity and lasts from days to weeks, this is referred to as post-exertional malaise. When you are setting goals and progressing with physical activity in all areas, it is important to identify an amount and intensity that does not worsen your symptoms after the activity, or in the days following. This can take a little trial and error and that is fine. Remember, the aim is for longer-term progress and consistency. If post-exertional malaise is an experience you can relate to, it is important that you consider activities that reduce the chances or the severity of this happening in the future so you can continue to tolerate, enjoy and make gradual progress in your physical activity. When the fatigue after physical exertion sets you back a few days, this can be demoralising and feel like a setback. Remember, it is normal to feel this way.

> *'I am much better now in terms of walking and running. I put this down to regular shortish walks and some low-paced short runs. In terms of other developments, I have limited the time spent on heavy tasks so as not to fall into the exhaustion zone and ruin the following day's activities. I have also maintained my ability to drive long distances by starting off with short journeys and increasing the distance.'*

Plan your daily activity to ensure that you are not pushing beyond the limits of your current energy levels. Think about your rate of perceived exertion (RPE) – see the box overleaf to get familiar with this. It is a simple way to figure out how hard you are exerting yourself by scoring this from zero to ten. Zero is the score for no exertion at all, and ten is the score for the maximum effort you can give. It can help you choose what activities to do as you progress in your recovery. These could include household chores, gardening, walking, swimming, cycling or whatever activities you have identified as important to you.

Borg CR10 scale*

Classification	Descriptor
0	Nothing at all
0.5	Very, very light
1	Very light
2	Fairly light
3	Moderate
4	Somewhat hard
5	Hard
6	-
7	Very hard
8	-
9	-
10	Very, very hard (maximum)

Please be aware that this is not the same as the 0–10 scale of fatigue following activity introduced in chapter 2, Managing Fatigue. The RPE in this chapter demonstrates a rating of *exertion* (how hard you feel you are working) *during* the physical activity, not the *fatigue after* physical activity.

We suggest that, to start with, you keep your RPE at 4 out of 10 or less, which is described as 'somewhat hard'. Practically, this is a level where you can make conversation while exerting yourself, although your breathing may be a little faster. You are still within your comfort zone, but you are working harder than usual. You could then monitor your symptoms to see how you respond to this.

---

* Borg, G., *Borg's perceived exertion and pain scales* (Human Kinetics, 1998).

'At the beginning of June there was a day where I woke up and suddenly felt the need to exercise. I started small with one 20-minute cycle per week and felt amazing afterwards. This progressed (while being mindful that I didn't want to overdo it again) to two then three times a week, and I have managed to maintain this ever since. I recognise that I needed to get to a place where I had enough energy to exercise, but in doing so it has given me more energy.'

If you experience significant post-exertional malaise, you should rest and recover, which means ensuring you have good hydration, nutrition, and both physical and mental rest. This is also a chance to reset the amount of energy you expend the next time. Take a note of whether you recover to pre-exertion levels an hour or so after physical activity, and also how you feel the next day. If you experience post-exertional malaise, this is a sign that you need to reset your level of exertion to a lower level for the next time.

Please also have a read through chapter 2, Managing Fatigue, which provides lots of really helpful guidance on how to manage your energy throughout a day by understanding energy requirements for tasks and monitoring how much you exert yourself when you're doing them.

Exercise in the highly physically active

In our clinic, we have met several athletes, and you may be able to relate their experience of Long Covid to your own. Prior to becoming unwell with Covid, you may have been very fit and training at a high level to compete in marathons and triathlons, for example. This might have required you to train regularly and intensely, often several times a week. Despite this, even very physically active and fit people can suffer with the debilitating symptoms of Long Covid, so much so that they may not be able to walk half a mile before having to stop. You may also have been left extremely fatigued following exercise, even for some days after, which may leave you feeling low and frustrated.

The best approach we have found for returning to physical activity for previously highly physically active people – and those not as physically active – is a symptom-guided return to physical activity. This is not as regimented as a 'graded return to training' schedule that some very physically active people and athletes are used to.

Recovery is vital following exercise in highly physically active people and optimising this can provide huge benefits to allow you to build and progress. The purpose is for your body and mind to have time to adapt and restore, to allow you to feel rejuvenated and ready to go again. There is much more to it than rest. Good quality and duration of sleep is vitally important, as is a nutritious diet containing enough calories to match your energy requirements and good hydration. Pay as much attention to your recovery as you do to your physical activity to progress in the best way possible.

You might be accustomed to using a wearable wrist device to track, analyse and record your step count, sleep patterns and heart rate when exercising. In many people who have had Covid, these measurements become less well controlled and more variable for a while. Using these devices can often cause worry and confusion, which can muddy the picture as you can't interpret them in the same way you did before being unwell. It is important to base how much you do on 1) how you *feel* when undertaking physical activity and 2) how well you *recover* afterwards. From our experience in helping people become more physically active, we have found that it is the symptoms and how you feel, rather than the numbers, that are best in providing guidance for progress. Many people we have helped have felt less anxious and more in tune with their body when exercising after they placed their devices and fitness apps aside for a while.

'I have found my fitness and strength levels gradually and consistently improving. The discipline of mindfulness and yoga exercises has given me a much better active awareness and perception of the level of exertion I am working at, rather than relying on my rather erratic heart rate on an activity tracker. Previously, my efforts to pace myself using heart rate as a marker of exertion hadn't been getting me anywhere. Not focusing on this has allowed me to continue building fitness at a sustainable level, which continues to gradually improve over time. This increase has also helped me continue to feel huge gratitude for the level of health and fitness I do currently have, and I feel more positive that I can continue to build this slow and sustained improvement to engage in the activities that I enjoy.'

TIPS FOR GETTING BACK ON TRACK

In addition to using the rate of perceived exertion (RPE) scale described earlier, you may find it helpful to consider the following useful tips and reminders to get yourself back on track:

- **Take your time.** Don't expect to return immediately. It will take time. Try not to compare yourself to how fit and active you felt you were before. Instead, compare yourself to how you were last week.

- **There is only one YOU.** There are large variations between individual athletic people in ability and time frame of response to physical activity with Long Covid. This means that the amount, intensity and progression is individual to you. Try your best not to compare your progress with that of other people affected by Long Covid – everyone has their own journey.

- **Listen to your body.** Covid can affect multiple organs in your body and recovery can be complicated. In athletes recovering from certain injuries, we may recommend increasing training loads by a certain percentage every week. However, these general rules do not really apply to those affected by Long Covid. For your progress in recovery, the increments may be adjusted by setting much smaller percentages or remaining at the same level for several weeks. You could use the RPE scale to help you see how you are doing and remain at a certain intensity until that activity is scored lower (easier) on the RPE scale. This could be the right time to make a small step in the duration or the intensity of the exercise – it is best not to change both at the same time as it becomes trickier to assess your progress or pin down what might cause setbacks, should they occur. We would recommend that you maintain the duration of an activity at the same RPE for a period of 2–3 weeks to establish a sustainable level before increasing the intensity of the exercise. Once you have built a foundation of aerobic endurance by doing aerobic exercise consistently at RPE 4 out of 10, this is the stage when you could consider exercise of a higher intensity.

- **Recovery is vital.** Following a day of greater than usual levels of physical activity, recovery might take longer than you were once used to or would like. Sleep forms a vital part of recovery and can provide a foundation for building your levels of physical activity. Replenish yourself through a healthy balanced diet and make sure you stay well hydrated.
- **Ask for support.** If you are a member of a sports club, we recommend that coaches and support staff familiarise themselves with Long Covid and how it can affect your current limitations as well as your goals. This will allow for any progress plans to be reviewed and perhaps rewritten, based on your expectations and abilities. Involve your exercise network – this might include friends, family or colleagues.
- **Be open to adjusting what you do.** It's a good idea to vary the intensity, length or type of exercise to allow longer periods for rest and recovery when you feel that you may have pushed yourself too much. Think about how you might cross-train with different types of aerobic exercises by choosing to switch between activities such as running, cycling or using a cross-trainer.
- **Be kind to yourself.** It's normal to feel tired, weak, unmotivated, anxious or depressed with Long Covid. You will have good days and bad days. Try not to get too low with the lows or too high with the highs. Make time for yourself. Accept these days as part of the process.

'I found it very challenging at first to adhere to what felt to me like such a "dialled back" programme, and which at first felt like going backwards rather than forwards. Ironically, trusting this much slower process needed more discipline and self-control than following my own inclination to push harder at every stage to get back to fitness! By sticking to the schedule and integrating complementary elements such as strength training and breath control through specialised yoga classes, I was able to avoid the "boom and bust" pattern and the post-exercise payback "crashes" that I had been experiencing before.'

Physical activity after deconditioning following Covid

When you were first affected by symptoms of Covid, you may have had a time in hospital or at home with bed rest and very little activity. This can often leave people feeling weak. Bed rest can significantly reduce muscle mass, muscle strength, aerobic fitness and physical function. This is referred to as deconditioning and can lead to loss in independence in carrying out everyday tasks. Deconditioning can make previously simple activities such as washing, dressing, walking or climbing stairs challenging.

Your symptoms may be fairly distressing and have a real impact on your everyday life. For that reason, it is important to be aware of how physical activity can make a real difference. This may help you have greater confidence to keep things up. Increased physical activity could make you feel less tired, and over time everyday tasks and activities may become a little easier. Here are some of the things that physical activity does for people who have become deconditioned after having had Covid:

- Helps keep the mind and brain working well.
- Improves muscle strength.
- Improves your ability to perform day-to-day activities.
- Improves your mobility and walking.
- Enhances mood and well-being.

You might really want to be more physically active but perhaps not know where to start. Do your best not to be judgemental or disappointed, no matter how little you do – any activity is better than no activity at all. It is useful to look at what you might typically do during a day or a week, and to explore where you might fit in some physical activity. Look for opportunities where you can reduce the amount of time being sedentary and increase the amount of time being active. This could involve simple changes, such as getting off the bus one stop before you usually do to allow you to have a short walk, using the stairs instead of the escalator, or standing up for a short walkabout at home during the advert breaks when watching the television. Be creative. Look for windows of opportunity to move more.

'During my recovery period I used body weight exercises then moved on to light weights, with the weights becoming heavier as I progressed. Although I still have health issues that are not yet resolved, I now feel more like a normal person who is not quite fully fit.'

Aim for your activities to be of moderate intensity – you can refer to the rate of perceived exertion (RPE) scale described earlier (see p. 92) [see italicised]. This would be a 4 out of 10 on the RPE scale. For most people, this will mean that you will experience a slightly faster breathing rate than usual, and you may feel that your heart is working more than it would normally. You are working harder, but within your comfort zone.

It is normal for anyone who is not used to being physically active to experience some muscle soreness after doing a new exercise. This does not mean that the activity has caused any damage, as it is a normal part of adapting to the increased work the muscles have done. As you become accustomed to the activity, this pain will usually reduce. Many of those who have musculoskeletal pain find that being more active helps to reduce their pain, as stronger muscles help to better support their joints.

If you have experienced deconditioning, keep in mind the following tips:
- Make a start! Anything is better than nothing.
- Start slowly and build up gradually – ask yourself, 'What's the easiest thing I could start with?'
- Try to do a variety of physical activity (aerobic, strength, balance and flexibility exercises) – these all have their own benefits.
- At home, aim to gradually build up to 30 minutes of activity per day, along with muscle strengthening and balance activities twice a week.
- Do what you enjoy!
- Being active with others can be great for keeping you motivated – who might you do this with?

LM is a 19-year-old personal trainer who came to the Long Covid clinic with symptoms that had affected her for several months. Have a read-through the interview to get an insight into her experience.

What were your concerns about physical activity before you went to the Long Covid clinic?

Being a personal trainer and student who was active, fit and very healthy, I was completely taken aback to find out what I thought would be an easy and fast recovery was in fact a slow and sometimes demotivating process. To begin with, it affected the small things like getting to college. I normally walked this, an hour each way, in the morning and evening. It set me up for the day and prepared me for my lessons. Due to the development of my symptoms, which persisted, the idea of walking such a long way didn't appeal to me and it was something I dreaded. I began to take taxis one way and try my best to walk the other. Not being able to participate in the sport that I love affected my confidence. Having been an enthusiastic, happy, motivated 19-year-old, I soon turned into what I thought was a lazy, boring and uninspired individual with nothing left. About six months after I contracted Covid, I realised I was so unhappy and just couldn't be bothered to do normal day-to-day things, like walk the dog. This put me off everything and the fear of not being able to do what I used to be able to do on a daily basis was a nightmare.

How were your expectations and targets affected after discussion at the clinic?

When I attended the Long Covid clinic I was still in a state of 'I don't want to', 'I can't do it', 'I hate everything to do with exercise'. Attending was hard for me because I was genuinely lost. I was asked to think about what I would say to my clients that I personal train, when they are just starting exercise after a long period of inactivity. I realised that I needed to stop being harsh on myself and that it was OK to take time.

What kind of plan did you discuss and how did you get on?

The first thing we agreed on was to take things slowly. Not expecting too much but also trying to get back into the habit of doing things without thinking about it. I started by doing scheduled walking and morning exercises, which were mainly yoga related, and I got into the habit of taking the dogs out twice a day. In a few weeks I started a higher-level intensity training, again every other day, rather than the 3–4 sessions a day that I used to lead my clients through in the gym before I became unwell with Covid. When I felt comfortable within my level of exertion, I started to do a slightly higher intensity, but ensuring that if my body didn't feel up to it, not to push myself because that would affect me more after the workout.

Did you face challenges in your progress and if so, what were they?
Challenges are inevitable, no one is the same. Lack of motivation is normal – everyone suffers from it sometimes. Some aches and pains are also more common and are part of the process when getting back into doing exercises that you have not done for a while. Doing my best not to judge myself was the key. I can't stress that enough. My main challenge was motivation, I was so nervous about not being able to do what I used to and people judging me. No one was judging me. The only person judging me was myself and this is something I became aware of as being something that would hold me back.

Where are you now in your physical activity and progress?
I now don't even think about the past. I do think about how far I've come, rather than why I can't do things any more. I train around 4–5 times a week and do yoga exercises most mornings. My training sessions previously were no longer than 40 minutes. Now they are more like 20 minutes, but still working with a good ratio of work for 40 seconds and rest for 20 seconds. I started from the bottom and worked up. An idea of mine was to use someone else to help motivate me. I am a personal trainer and love to make my own workouts. Soon, I realised that the workouts I was constructing were too hard, so I decided that I should let someone else do the work to help me stay within limits. I watched live guided exercise videos every time I worked out and loved it and got my mum and one of my friends to join me in the mornings, too. I am by no means completely back to how I used to be, but I am so much happier and feel that my recovery has been down to that one chat from the Covid clinic.

SUMMARY

- Be present – the starting point is where you are now. You can then look forward to progress.

- It is important to remember that you are not alone – there are many other people feeling low, frustrated, and looking for ways to recover, just like you.

- As you recover, you will learn to listen to your body to help you find the right balance between rest and activity.

- Setting goals can help you keep focused and motivated – keep them SMART.

- Look for signs of post-exertional malaise – keep a diary and adjust your levels of activity accordingly.

- Plan your daily activity to ensure that you are not pushing beyond the limits of your energy levels – think about your rate of perceived exertion (RPE).

- The best approach is a symptom-guided return to physical activity – focus on how you feel rather than focusing on numbers.

CHAPTER 6
Psychological Considerations

Until 2020, most of us had come to see infectious illness like the flu or common cold as an inevitable, albeit inconvenient part of life that we didn't need to worry about too much. The Covid pandemic, let's face it, hasn't been like this at all. It's been, and continues to be, frightening. Having any illness has a psychological impact; those that require self-management can be particularly demanding. In this chapter we consider some of the psychological challenges that may arise when you have Long Covid and identify variables that can be useful to address to support you in your journey towards recovery. Lastly, drawing from techniques that many patients have found helpful, a psychologically focused self-help approach is laid out that integrates with practical advice from the other chapters.

The many questions surrounding Covid

Being unwell with a flu-like virus is at the best of times inconvenient and annoying, but the symptoms are familiar to us – congestion, aches and pains, fatigue. Mostly we put up with them and wait to get better. A bit of worry might start to creep in if things don't go as expected, and we may find ourselves wondering – When will I get better? What if this gets worse? Do I need to take time off? Do I need to rest? Feedback from others is often welcome at this point – 'you'll be fine in a few days', 'take it easy', 'it's just a cold' – and mostly we feel reassured. If symptoms do carry on longer than expected or new ones appear, we know there is someone at hand to help, whether the family doctor or pharmacist perhaps, who will be able to make sense of things and get us on the right track. Mostly, though, it's all familiar and we're confident we'll get better because that's what's happened before.

With Covid, we haven't had the usual reassurance – in fact, quite the opposite. Doctors and scientists have been desperately trying to work out the answers to so many questions – Who is at risk? What are the symptoms? How infectious is it? How do we keep ourselves safe? Do we recover like we do from a cold, or are there long-term consequences for our health? At one time or another, most of us are likely to have asked ourselves: Will I be OK? Will I survive if I get Covid? You are likely to have been afraid for others, and maybe for yourself, before you got Covid. After contracting Covid, even if you had just a few mild symptoms, you are likely to have been concerned as we know symptoms can get worse quickly, some aren't easy to notice, and we are advised to monitor ourselves, take our temperature, think about our breathing, buy a pulse oximeter and monitor oxygen saturations. You may have wondered at times – Is it getting worse? Am I going to need urgent care? Am I going to get the care I need at the right time? Am I going to survive this? Many people have been very unwell with Covid and may have required hospital admission. For others, life and death may have hung in the balance for themselves or their loved ones. Wherever you have been on the spectrum of illness, you are likely to have been concerned and sat with high levels of uncertainty. Covid, it is fair to say, has been traumatic.

However badly you had Covid, treating the acute illness is the part the doctors now know the most about. Although there is still research being undertaken about the best treatments for acute Covid infection, there have been advances that significantly improve prognosis from severe Covid. However, if you caught Covid early on, you wouldn't have had the reassurance that you were necessarily getting the right treatment.

Expectations following Covid-19 infection

So, the good news – you have recovered from your acute illness, and from a medical perspective this is where things end. You can get back to life as normal and although it might take a bit of time, you are going to get back to where you were, just like you did when you were ill with a cold or the flu.

But for many people, yourself probably included, this hasn't happened. You may have had a period when you felt like you'd got your mojo back or were 'nearly there', or you may have found that your symptoms lingered on and on and things just haven't improved. They may even have got worse. For many, it is the physical and/or mental tiredness and breathlessness that is the major problem, but there are many other symptoms that may have carried on from when you were unwell, or new ones that have emerged or appear from time to time, with no apparent rhyme or reason.

> 'After being unwell with Covid for a few weeks I got back to work, and started running again, I was feeling positive – I thought I had recovered, but then I started to feel unwell, and exhausted after exercise, I didn't know what was wrong – I was really worried.'

You might have tried to find out what was going on, and asked yourself: Why am I still unwell? Why am I unwell again? You may have turned to your doctor or looked online in an attempt to find out. Unfortunately, the world of medicine doesn't do well with symptoms and problems that it doesn't have a label for, and if you saw your doctor early in the pandemic (or even recently), you may have felt your doctor didn't know what was wrong.

> 'My GP said my headaches weren't related to having had Covid, and when I eventually saw a specialist they said the same. I felt at a loss, like I was making it up because I'd not had headaches like this before. Then I read online that lots of people with Long Covid are also experiencing headaches like mine, and I felt angry and let down.'

Long Covid of course isn't (or hasn't been) in the doctors' compendiums of illness and conditions. If you have seen a doctor about your symptoms, it is quite possible they were unsure or even came across as dismissive. If they did, this is unlikely to have helped and many people with Long Covid report feeling frustrated, angry, hopeless or just stuck after they've seen a doctor. Unfortunately, there are still many gaps in our knowledge and questions to be answered, so to be left feeling despairing after a medical appointment isn't that unusual (it's frustrating, but doctors are usually trying their best to help, within the established knowledge that they have). From the perspective of your well-being, however, this is a big problem – however worried you felt before you went to see the doctor, this has now got a whole lot worse. If the doctors don't even know what's wrong, how can they help? What does that mean for me? Am I on my own with this? Will I ever get better? Has Covid caused permanent damage? These are very distressing thoughts to sit with, and it is not surprising that many people with Long Covid feel anxious, hopeless and low in mood.

It can be helpful to remember that there are lots of symptoms – aches, pains, occasional irregularities of one body system or another – that aren't a sign of any medical problem at all, and it is the doctor's job to try and work out which are serious and which are not. In fact, as much as 50 per cent of all reasons for visiting a GP concern symptoms that aren't caused by anything serious, and are likely to pass of their own accord. On a more positive note, things are improving as we learn more about the after-effects of Covid and many doctors now have a better understanding of Long Covid and can provide helpful guidance.

You may have had a difficult time getting your doctor to understand, but what about friends, family and colleagues? It can be hard for them to really fathom what is going on, too. You may be fortunate and have supportive people around you, but many of us don't and can be left feeling misunderstood and unsupported. You may have debilitating symptoms that are affecting your ability to do things you want or need to do, like work, go shopping, cook a meal, look after the children, socialise and exercise. You might have stopped, reduced or found a workaround for some things you used to do, or have no choice but to carry on despite your symptoms. It is natural to worry if your symptoms get worse, or you have little confidence that you'll get better – if medical professionals aren't providing any answers, it would be understandable for you to start looking elsewhere for things that are going to help. Lots of us will automatically turn to the internet and start looking at what comes up. There may be some degree of relief and reassurance provided, but also uncertainty about the best course of action – people telling their stories, giving advice and opinions, some reassuring, some not, some very worrying. What do you do? Should you rest? Should you not rest? Should you take a supplement or try a new, untested treatment? If so, for how long should you try it and what to do if you feel worse?

A lot of decisions and a lot of uncertainty about any course of action. Things can quickly start to become confusing and overwhelming, dealing with the impact of symptoms on your life, the advice (or lack of it) from others, and working out what will help you get better and what might make things worse. Put simply, lack of clarity about the cause of symptoms, your prognosis and course of treatment can make it extremely stressful living with Long Covid.

'I had multiple investigations, all of which were normal. This was reassuring but frustrating in equal measure as I still had no answers as to why I was feeling this way or how long it would last. People kept telling me, "You just need to rest and give it time", "It is going to get better", but how did they know that? This was a new virus, one that we were still learning about. I genuinely considered that this might be it for me now, this might be how I was going to feel forever.'

The psychological impact of dealing with Covid and Long Covid has and continues to be significant for many, but it isn't an area that gets as much attention as it should. Medicine and healthcare systems across the world have a tendency to treat the mind and body as separate entities, rarely interacting. Our experience working in Long Covid is that taking a more integrated perspective is often very helpful, enabling the development of individual treatment plans. The aim of this chapter is to raise awareness of the possible contribution of psychological factors in Long Covid, and most importantly, to share some of the approaches and strategies patients have found to be helpful.

Stress and illness

The stress you feel when you are going to be late, have a test or interview coming up, or when you are in danger, is different to the kind of stress you can get with Long Covid – the first type of stress GOES AWAY sooner or later. Things calm down, you get through it, maybe you miss the appointment, or didn't even end up being late, but you relax eventually. Long Covid, on the other hand, is long term and symptoms and uncertainties are ongoing; there isn't any respite.

Most of us have heard that stress isn't good for us – and generally, this is about right. In reality, however, getting stressed from time to time can be very useful. It helps you to get things done, make it to an appointment on time, or fight off a crocodile, that sort of thing, but mostly it isn't good for us when it sticks around long term. You may have come across terms like stress-induced headache or even stress-induced heart attack. In fact, long-standing or chronic stress is linked to numerous health problems, including obesity, diabetes, cardiac disease, indigestion, back problems, sexual problems, and irritable bowel syndrome (stomach issues). The stress of heartbreak is even thought to cause a small number of deaths each year (called Takotsubo cardiomyopathy or broken heart syndrome, caused by a surge of stress hormones).

Stress is well known to have a lot of negative effects on the body. Some of the most well-recognised consequences are:

- headache and migraine;
- comfort eating – craving sweet and fatty foods;
- increased blood pressure;
- rashes, cold sores or ulcers;
- reduced sex drive;
- disturbed sleep at night;
- reduced concentration;
- forgetfulness;
- digestive problems (e.g. nausea, bloating, cramps and diarrhoea);
- fatigue.

It can be difficult to know if stress, whether due to being unwell or from other areas of your life, is playing a role in your illness. It can help to keep an open mind about it, though. When we are stressed a lot of the time, we can get so used to it that we stop recognising that it is even there. This could be an important part of the jigsaw puzzle – there is unlikely to be much to lose by taking some time to consider it, and it could be an area you have a degree of control over. It might help reduce the burden of symptoms.

Chronic stress, the sort that sticks around, is known to be pretty bad for us and it doesn't make us feel good either. It causes us, among many things, to feel tired and irritable, interferes with sleep, and promotes muscle tightness (often around the shoulders/neck). Stress can make us more alert to danger and makes it difficult to relax. If you are already unwell, especially with something that has made you fatigued and weak, the last thing your body needs is to get stressed. But unfortunately, it is completely natural for this to happen in chronic illness, especially Long Covid, where there is so much uncertainty. We know, especially in long-term health conditions, that stress can make symptoms worse, contribute to new ones, and may even get in the way of recovery.

It might seem far-fetched, and it would be understandable if you don't feel this applies to you, but research backs this up. Ever had a cold that doesn't go away? Or known someone who seems to get colds a lot? Ever noticed that you or they were going through a busy time or there was a lot going on? You might not say you are stressed, maybe just under pressure, but your body doesn't care about terminology. Put simply, stress can get in the way of your body healing. Healing may be slower, much slower, or may not even happen at all.

Biologically, there is substantial evidence to indicate that stress suppresses our immune system. Doctors used to think of the immune system as a completely separate biological system – running in the background, no matter the circumstances, serving to fight infection and keep us well. This has been found time and time again simply not to be true. Shift workers who have disturbed sleep, those who eat a lot of highly processed foods and people with post-traumatic stress disorder, to name a few examples, are known to have weakened immune systems and are more vulnerable to illness. Do we know stress definitely plays a role in Long Covid? No we don't. It probably isn't relevant for everyone with Long Covid, but it is worth considering based on what we know about other health conditions.

Doctors know that stress can interfere with medical problems – but it's a tricky subject. If a doctor does mention stress or anxiety, in an often too brief appointment, you can very easily feel that you are not being taken seriously, and that 'it's all in your head'. This is a horrid place to be, and quite rightly it causes many people to feel angry. Unfortunately, it could also mean you are more careful about discussing anything other than your physical symptoms again with a medical professional. Often, busy doctors might choose to skip the subject entirely. If you have been told, or it's been implied, that it's all psychological, and therefore by implication not real, just remember they are wrong – you are not making this up, these are real symptoms that need to be taken seriously.

Identifying and reducing stress can be one of the most important things you can do to help yourself when you are ill, but an issue you are still sadly least likely to get help with identifying and managing.

The stress of being unwell with Long Covid can be overwhelming enough, but life circumstances can also have a big impact on how difficult it is coping with being unwell. If you've got a lot of demands on you, such as caring responsibilities, and have little time to yourself, or if you've been through a lot of stressful life events, you may be more vulnerable to higher levels of stress. Feeling unsupported, or uncared for, during a time of illness is likely to increase stress further. Some of us aren't good at letting people know we are unwell. We don't want to burden those around us or let anyone down; we ignore how we are feeling and try to carry on with a smile on our face. This reaction and way of coping can lead to a lot of problems. People don't know how you are feeling and expectations remain in place. Furthermore, it means you can't do the things that are likely to help you get better, like pacing yourself and relaxing/resting. You are likely to feel increasingly alone, isolated with your suffering, exhausted and worn out as you try and carry on. Being able to talk through difficulties, share uncertainties and get practical help has a soothing, de-stressing effect, and can allow you to start to make the practical changes that help support recovery.

'The kids were not aware of the gulf between how I thought our family should be versus how things actually were because of my health. That was my sadness and grieving, not theirs. I needed to often remind myself of this.'

Adjusting to being unwell

For some of us, the way we manage our internal and external world, and what may work very well for us when we are in good health does not help, or even starts working against us, when we are unwell with a chronic health condition. It can be worth taking some time to think about ways in which you approach things in your life that may no longer be so helpful now you are unwell.

There are many different sorts of adjustments that people have found helpful to make with Long Covid and it is not possible to mention them all in this chapter. We have found in this clinic that many people maintain high standards for themselves, and are or aspire to be high achievers. This might relate to a few or a lot of areas of life (e.g. work, home life or relationships); you may feel that things need to be done a certain way or to a certain timescale. It is worth considering: do you need to make sure the kitchen is completely tidy before you can relax? Or make sure an email hasn't got any errors in before you send it? Are you juggling many important responsibilities and worry about dropping 'one of the balls'? Do you focus completely on getting the job done, and forget that you need to take a break or have something to eat? Examples such as these are signs that you might be someone with high standards. Is this really a problem? It can be very rewarding to do things well and be busy and productive. Many successful people talk positively about how doing this has helped them go far in life. The problem is, these behaviours can mean that you don't listen to your body, or ignore it completely, and so you don't do some of the things you need to do to get better. In fact, you might push yourself so much that you get more unwell as a consequence, only finally stopping when symptoms are really bad – when you are literally on the floor.

> 'As a nurse, I have been conditioned to work hard. Constantly thinking about the quickest and most efficient way of managing multiple tasks, all the while putting patients' needs above my own. I love my vocation, but the word "lazy" is often thrown around in a derogatory way and I was determined to prove that I was not "just tired" or "being lazy". I was conscious that people appeared to be fed up with my response when asked, "How are you?" and I didn't want to be perceived as a "moaner", so I tried my hardest to pretend that I was fine, until I wasn't.'

Psychologists and others sometimes use the word 'perfectionism' to describe this trait when things get extreme – it may be something you or others have identified in you, and it can be useful to consider ways in which it might have a negative impact on your well-being and on how you look after yourself. Are you constantly striving to do things to the very best of your ability? Do you often feel things aren't good enough? Does everything feel important? Do you get stressed over small things? Do you struggle to cope when things are uncertain? Do you feel dissatisfied a lot of the time? Being a 'perfectionist' can be seen as a badge of honour – 'my only flaw!', as people sometimes say in job interviews. It can mean, though, that self-managing symptoms like fatigue, and coping with the uncertainty of Long Covid, can be particularly difficult. It can make resting, relaxing and other self-management actions harder to do. Perfectionism can become a chronic stressor. We also know from research that it can contribute to mental health problems, meaning you are prone to anxiety and low mood, and help from a mental health practitioner like a psychologist can help in recognising and managing beliefs and behaviours that drive perfectionism and support you in developing strategies that make life easier to manage.

'Changing/lowering my standards helped give me the recovery time I needed. Learning to accept that my body wasn't up to doing the cleaning in the same way as when I was well was difficult, but ultimately helpful. I'm not sure I need to go back to doing things as well as I did them before.'

Blind and silent stress

Psychologists think that, over time, being in stressful circumstances and keeping negative thoughts and feelings to ourselves can be damaging to our mental and physical health. We rarely get the opportunity to stop and question things in life, and mostly we get used to, adapt to and cope as best we can with the circumstances we find ourselves in. Sometimes, though, you are in an environment that is unhealthy and stressful, but perhaps like a frog who doesn't notice the temperature rising in the pot they've found themselves in, you too haven't noticed – you are in many ways 'blind' to the stress you are in. It may only be feedback from others that alerts you to this possibility. Or, you are well aware that circumstances are difficult, and you know they are having a negative impact on your well-being, but perhaps because you feel you can't change things, or that talking about it will make you feel worse, you stay silent. Below are some common blind and silent stressors:

- Working in unreasonable conditions with excessively long hours, too much pressure, not enough support, or difficult or abusive colleagues and/or managers.
- Caring for children with emotional, behavioural or health problems.
- Being in an unhappy relationship, especially if you live with someone who makes you feel bad about yourself, is manipulative, uncompassionate or is simply not able to meet your emotional needs.

- Feeling on edge as a result of past trauma and seeing this as the norm.
- Living with lots of guilt or shame – feeling that you are constantly letting yourself or others down.

It can be useful to consider whether pressures such as these are present in your life. It is often very difficult to acknowledge that they are even there, and talking with an impartial friend or mental health professional can be helpful. Many of these issues are unlikely to be easy or even possible to address or resolve; often though there can be considerable benefit in recognising them and gaining the support and empathy of others.

> 'The appointment with the psychologist helped me recognise what was going on and I started putting things in place afterwards. I've seen quite an improvement since the first appointment.'

Mental health

The pain, suffering and debilitating effects of symptoms can have a very damaging effect on your mood, and lead to depression and anxiety. A lower mood can mean you get less pleasure from life and you might feel like doing less. You may find that you experience more negative thoughts about yourself and your future. Anxiety can also stop you wanting to do things and cause you to feel more isolated, which in turn can contribute to a lower mood.

> 'I was stressed and fatigued to the point of being unable to find words or spell. I was terrified that I was going to make a mistake, and again had to be signed off. This had a detrimental impact on my mental health. I felt like a failure.'

Many people find that their mood naturally improves once they start seeing an improvement in symptoms, but for others it is more complicated. The pandemic has affected people's lives in many negative ways, such as causing financial hardship, and isolation due to the effects of lockdowns. If you have had problems with your health in the past that have been traumatic or had experiences that have been particularly painful or difficult in childhood or later in life – what psychologists refer to as 'adverse events' – then managing your symptoms associated with Long Covid could be more difficult. Covid and Long Covid can trigger psychological trauma. Old coping strategies that have got you through past difficulties, such as pushing through or not asking for help, might not work as well now. Sometimes we find that people who have experienced a lot of trauma find it particularly difficult to take proper care of themselves when they are unwell; for example, they find it difficult to relax, pace and adjust expectations of themselves. Similarly, if you've struggled with worry or health anxiety in the past, it would be understandable if the experience of having Covid and Long Covid has made it worse.

Managing and recovering from Long Covid – next steps

For many people who are overwhelmed by the debilitating symptoms of Long Covid, not having a clear idea of how to manage those symptoms, or knowing if or when they will get better, is a huge problem. The advice below is offered to help you manage your symptoms and assist in your journey to recovery. This is the advice we give to patients with Long Covid – although, of course, in clinic all advice is tailored to individual circumstances and some or all advice may not be appropriate to your specific symptoms and circumstances.

1. Remember – you can recover from Long Covid

People are recovering from Long Covid. Many are seeing improvements in their symptoms and have been able to return to work, study and leisure activities (even discover new ones). We are seeing people getting back to exercise and beginning to enjoy life again. You will have your own trajectory, and for some people it is a slow, difficult process and is taking a long time. Don't let yourself be consumed by negative opinions, unsubstantiated claims or bad science that takes a pessimistic view of your prognosis. If you are finding that particular sources of information make you feel more worried about your Long Covid, reduce or stop your exposure to them. Seek out positive personal stories of recovery – there are many out there, so remember this can and will be you.

'It took a long time and a lot of work but 13 months from onset, it felt as if the cloud had lifted. I had more energy, my headaches had completely disappeared, and as long as I didn't allow myself to get fatigued the brain fog and fevers were more manageable.'

2. Put a recovery programme in place

One of the most effective ways to feel more positive about getting better is to put a practical recovery plan in place. This will work best if it is tailored to your specific circumstances and symptoms – the principles of chapters 2 and 5 should help you get started with putting this together, but guidance from a Long Covid specialist may be needed to get this right for you. It will focus on helping you to gain control over the most problematic symptoms. Getting the philosophy of recovery right can be important – you may come across contradictory advice online or from other sources, on the one hand suggesting you 'listen to your body' and do as you feel, and on the other saying you need to stick to a strict pattern of activity/exercise and rest, push through symptoms, and not really listen to your body at all. Most people who make good progress find that neither position, when taken to an extreme, is helpful; it is often about finding the right balance between these two approaches – and that can take time. The majority of people we see find that focusing sensitively on managing the three key parts of life (activity/ work, rest and sleep) are the main building blocks of their recovery.

Remember, you might not get your recovery plan right to begin with – you may need to move things around, and it is not uncommon for people to be too ambitious to start with and find that symptoms get worse rather than better. Don't give up: it may take some time to find the right starting point.

Monitor your progress on your recovery plan and check off items at the end of each day at least. Review your progress at the end of each week: Was it about right? Do you need to make a change? Can you increase things?

'Things have got better and anxiety has reduced. Seeing progress has reduced my anxiety, and I feel more confident about getting better over the longer term. I've been exercising regularly over the past couple of months now, and feeling generally, day-to-day better. Getting back to work has helped.'

3. Start a relaxation activity and do it daily

Prioritise relaxation. Regular relaxation can have many benefits, including improving concentration, mood, sleep and digestion and reducing muscle tension, pain and negative emotions. Give yourself regular time each day to relax – ideally, two sessions a day of at least 15 minutes. Relaxation should help you feel calm, settled and safe; ideally you will be focusing on the here and now, away from thoughts or images that take you into the past or future. If you have a tried-and-tested relaxation or mediation technique, now is the time to use it – it might be a mindfulness exercise, a religious meditation, a belly-breathing exercise, or a progressive muscular relaxation exercise. It could be stroking a pet, focusing on a tree or clouds, or using your imagination to put you in a safe and relaxing place.

You want your heart rate and your breathing to slow – you are, in physiological terms, activating your parasympathetic nervous system and entering into a biological state of rest, and with it safety. It might be that you don't tend to really relax, that it is difficult or even uncomfortable when you do so, or that you feel the things you already do are good enough, like watching TV, playing games online, or chatting. I would urge you to think again. The world we live in tends not to encourage us to use our leisure time to engage in proper, deep relaxation – these other activities are a nice break, and can be very enjoyable, but they are unlikely to promote the same quality of relaxation as the activities suggested above. Give it a go! Bear in mind it is going to take a bit of work and determination to prioritise two periods of relaxation a day, and it will be a couple of weeks before you are able to tell if it is making a difference – the results are not going to be immediately obvious.

This could be an important part of your recovery and it will work much better if you assign a time each day to do it, rather than wait until you are very stressed or anxious. Remember, you are important – you need to find and dedicate time to yourself to get better. **Time spent relaxing isn't time wasted, it's time invested.**

'I wanted to make my rests as restorative as possible – this did NOT mean reading, scrolling, emailing, doing an online food shop while lying down, or listening. Restorative rest for me meant lying down with eyes closed, looking out of a window at clouds or trees,

silence or at least quiet, possibly listening to a meditation such as Headspace or Mindfulness App.'

4. Remember your path to recovery may not be smooth

Remaining hopeful is important in so many areas of life, but particularly when you are unwell with Long Covid. It is completely normal to feel frustrated and hopeless, especially if you have an increase in symptoms or just don't seem to be improving. Symptoms can flare up and sometimes we can identify the reasons for this, but at other times we can't. The path is rarely smooth, and it can be a very bumpy ride. The diagram below illustrates what many people with Long Covid describe about their illness journey – they hope and expect a steady recovery, but find it isn't like that at all – it can be beset with obstacles and challenges that each need a strategy to overcome. Although very hard to do, it is really important to remember that a setback does not mean you have gone backwards completely, or that you aren't going to get better. It can help illuminate a barrier or issue that needs to be addressed, and while problem solving can be helpful, at other times we may need to just accept that life is difficult right now. Variables outside of your control or that are unknowable might have caused the setback – but things will improve. You may need some help and support and temporarily to adjust your management plan.

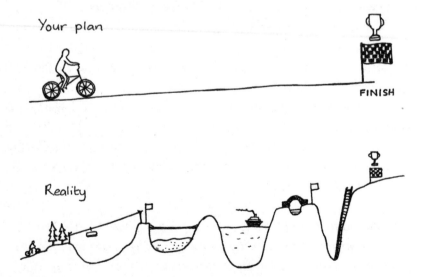

The plan versus the reality of getting to your goal.

5. Notice and celebrate improvements

Make sure you notice improvements in symptoms, or in what you are achieving. Those who make the most sustained recovery tend to make progress gradually. This means it can be easy not to notice or to dismiss these changes. Remember, small changes are meaningful – lots of small steps soon add up to a long distance travelled. Noticing and celebrating improvements will help to improve your mood, reduce anxiety and make you feel more positive about symptoms improving. Equally, it is important not to get carried away – noticing an improvement does not mean you are better and can abandon your recovery plan just yet.

> 'I'm looking after me now. I feel like I understand what is going on. The symptoms were very hard to deal with; the brain fog in particular and how it comes and goes. Keeping a diary, and being able to make some sense of symptoms has really helped. I no longer feel so low.'

6. Address mental health problems

The Covid pandemic has seen the number of people suffering with mental health problems soar. For many who had a pre-existing mental health condition, these difficulties have become worse. The impact of Long Covid symptoms on mental health is likely to be very significant indeed and we know that depression and anxiety are commonly reported by those who suffer with chronic physical symptoms.

If your mood is low, or you are very anxious, don't suffer alone – get help. Thankfully, these days there is a better appreciation of the pain and suffering that mental health problems cause, and efforts are ongoing to reduce the shame and stigma felt and experienced by many. Healthcare providers are used to talking to people about their mental health, but won't always ask you directly about it – it is OK to bring it up, to talk about how you are feeling. It is particularly important to seek help if you start having thoughts about harming yourself. The access to NHS mental health services in the UK has been improving, but still varies quite a bit according to where you live. Talking therapies are recommended as first line treatments for anxiety and depression, and can be highly effective, but an assessment by a suitably qualified mental health professional can help direct you to the services that are right for you. Often it is best to start with booking an appointment with your GP.

7. Practise saying 'no' and if possible be open and honest with those around you

If you are someone who doesn't like to let others know how you are feeling, you don't like to ask for help or you push yourself to do what you think you should do, you might be putting more strain on yourself, and this won't help you with your recovery. Try being open and honest with others about what you can manage: you may need to set boundaries, you may need to practise saying no. This can feel very uncomfortable, but people may be more understanding than you imagine and often don't even need an explanation for 'Sorry, I can't' or 'Would you be able to pick up the kids for me next week?' Remember, you don't always have to fully explain why you can't take on something new or need to step back from some of your responsibilities.

8. Reduce stressors in your life where possible

Are there things in your life that are causing a lot of stress? Is there anything you can do to minimise or remove them entirely?

Are your expectations of yourself too high? Are you pushing yourself too much to get things done or to achieve things to the same level or at the same speed as you did when you were well? If you have adjusted your expectations of yourself, have you adjusted them enough?

Are you taking too much responsibility for things in life? Can you delegate to someone else (think about the different domains of your life – home, work, family)? Can you focus just on what is really important, and leave the rest?

Is there a relationship in your life that is difficult to manage? Could you put boundaries in place with them (for example, how often you see or talk to them)? Or even tell them how you feel? Do some people need to know you have a health problem so they can support you?

It can feel important to be connected with current affairs, but the constant stream of negative news stories can fuel anxiety and stress. Consider consuming your preferred medium of news once a day, or less. Avoid checking the news on your phone; consider deleting news apps and turning off news notifications.

Are you sitting with a lot of negative emotions – for example, anger, frustration, fear, hopelessness, resentment, shame or guilt? If this is the case, speak to someone about it – this isn't easy, some things are extremely difficult to address and need careful professional support, whether that's via a voluntary or statutory organisation or a therapist. Your GP can help signpost you to sources of help. You can also look for a registered counsellor or psychologist yourself; in the UK, this will be someone registered with the HCPC (Health and Care Professions Council), although you will normally have to pay or use private health insurance.

'The first appointment was really important, I felt supported and understood, and that helped reduce my anxiety, feeling that someone knew what I was going through, and would be able to help me.'

9. Be careful monitoring symptoms

It is natural to pay attention to symptoms we are worried about, and often doctors encourage us to do exactly that. Unfortunately, this can also be worrying, and we can fall into a pattern of excessive monitoring or continuing to monitor a symptom after the doctors have told us we no longer need to do so. The easy availability of temperature, heart, sleep and other trackers can make it very tempting to do, even if it hasn't been advised. For some, this monitoring can keep health concerns 'alive'. Consider whether you really do need to keep up the monitoring and experiment with increasing your time away from it. You might feel more anxious to begin with, but over time your anxiety and focus on particular symptoms will hopefully reduce.

'In terms of heart rate monitoring watches, I wore one for a bit. The data it generated effectively told me I was not as well as I thought and occasionally it would vibrate and alarm rather disturbingly until I changed what I was doing. These were helpful messages to be reminded about, but after a few weeks I felt I understood its message of "go gently" and the smartwatch has long been abandoned in a box.'

SUMMARY

- The contribution of our mental health and our psychological make-up has long been acknowledged to play an important, often essential, role in determining how we cope with illness, and may be particularly important in chronic conditions where we have, to some degree, to take care of ourselves.

- Self-management appears to be important in Long Covid. Taking a psychologically informed approach may help provide you with the tools needed to navigate towards recovery.

- People are improving and getting better, but there does not appear to be a 'magic bullet'. In some ways, that is not surprising – we are all unique, each with a different social, environmental, biological and psychological make-up, and the contribution of these factors varies hugely from person to person. Taking an individualised approach that takes account of these factors is often the most helpful.

- Having Long Covid is likely to affect nearly everyone psychologically in one way or another, but reaching out, getting support and advice or simply having someone really listen can help you through difficult times.

'While I realise that I am still not where I was pre-Covid, I am not sure that I ever want to be. I now have perspective and respect for my body and health, both physically and mentally.'

CHAPTER 7
Managing Loss of Smell

Roughly half of all people in the UK who had Covid-19 have found them-selves with problems with smell and related loss of taste. This chapter has some practical tips and advice for helping you to manage this problem and give yourself the best chance of recovery.

What happened to my sense of smell?

The nose is one of the places in the body where the Covid virus can gain entry. The olfactory (from the Latin for 'to smell') nerves and specialised tissue high in the nasal passages are responsible for smell and link the smells in the atmosphere to our brain. For this reason, our sense of smell is already vulnerable to things in the environment like chemicals and smoke.

At present, it is not fully understood how SARS-CoV2, the virus causing Covid-19 infection, causes smell impairment, but scientists believe that it may relate to damage or inflammation to the olfactory nerves or the cells that support them. The good news is that these cells have the ability to repair themselves, and they do this well – but it takes time.

You might have lost your sense of smell very quickly, as if a switch turned it off. Some people noticed this before they had other symptoms; for others, it was during or after the initial illness. The way smell is affected by Covid can be different for each person. So, when you read about how others are affected, don't be concerned if your story isn't the same.

How long will it take to recover?

Within the group of people who have lost their sense of smell, we find two recovery patterns. In the first group, people recover quickly and completely, without further smell problems. We do not know why this happens, but

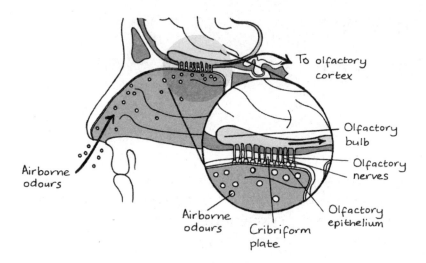

To olfactory cortex

Olfactory bulb

Olfactory nerves

Olfactory epithelium

Airborne odours

Airborne odours

Cribriform plate

This diagram shows how smells are detected. Odours are inhaled into our nose, which stimulates receptors on the olfactory nerve fibres situated at the top of our nasal cavity. This triggers electrical impulse along the nerve fibres to the olfactory bulb and to other areas of the brain that then interprets the smell. This pathway is disrupted by the SARS-CoV2 virus.

one possibility is that the virus causes localised inflammation and swelling high in the upper airway, behind the bridge of the nose. This swelling blocks the smell molecules from reaching the receptors that help the brain interpret odour. People in this first group have what is called 'conductive loss' of smell. The air can't get to the right place and the brain can't interpret any smell, so it's similar to pinching your nose closed. These people will regain smell quickly after the virus has cleared and the inflammation and swelling have settled, usually within a period of weeks. The vast majority of people who have lost their sense of smell with Covid are in this group.

For people in the second recovery group, something different is going on. Here, the virus is thought to enter and damage the cells that support the functioning of olfactory nerves. This means that the nerves are not able to do their job. After the virus has cleared, the damage remains. This damage can heal, but takes time. You will need patience during your recovery.

Many people ask: 'When will my sense of smell be 100 per cent again?' This is a natural question, and one that causes a great deal of anxiety, especially for people who are in the early stages of their smell loss. It is important to remember that this kind of nerve damage is like an injury, rather than something that you 'recover' from. Like a broken leg, it will take time – and nerve recovery is a slow process. However, there are ways that are scientifically proven to speed up this process, and we will discuss this later in the chapter.

So, recovery can follow one of two patterns: a fairly quick recovery within a couple of weeks, or a slower recovery pattern that might take over a year. Unfortunately, it is not possible to identify which group you might be in. Once you have been without smell for two months, it is reasonable to assume that your smell loss is related to damage to the olfactory nerve pathway.

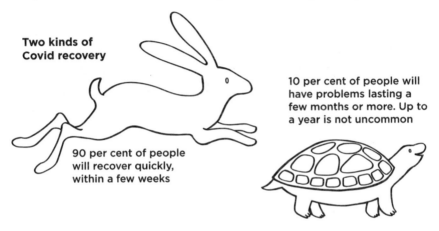

Two kinds of Covid recovery

10 per cent of people will have problems lasting a few months or more. Up to a year is not uncommon

90 per cent of people will recover quickly, within a few weeks

What is recovery like?

For the 90 per cent of people with no nerve damage, recovery will be swift and complete. These people will recover anyway, whether or not they load up on supplements to help their sense of smell or try smell training or any other remedies. It is important to point out that many of the 'cures' you read about on the internet are cases of people in this quick recovery group – because it can be so stressful to lose your sense of smell, people are often willing to 'try anything', and may attribute recovery to whatever 'treatment' they were trying nearest to the time their smell returned, even though their smell was destined to return by itself. Therefore, great care is needed when interpreting unsubstantiated claims that specific remedies can cure smell loss.

For people who take longer to recover, we see two different stories.

1. Some people experience a degree of recovery, and things smell 'normal'. In other words, their sense of smell might be weak, but the smells they do experience are what they would expect. This weak sense of smell is called *hyposmia*. Their sense of smell may remain this way for some time – how long is currently the subject of extensive research.

2. The second pattern of recovery includes 'qualitative changes' to the sense of smell.

- *Parosmia* is one of these. Parosmia means smells are altered, distorted, or even revolting. People describe the experience as being like smelling sewage, burning oil, spoiled meat or something sickly sweet. Very often it is accompanied by a sense of disgust. It is a trigger in the environment, such as food, that causes this experience.
- Another condition, known as *phantosmia*, is a constant background smell, often unpleasant, that has **not** been triggered by something in the environment. Parosmia and phantosmia often, but not always, occur together. Phantosmia can be likened to tinnitus – it's a sensory experience that originates in the brain, rather than in the real world.

Doctors and researchers are still learning about the longer-term outcomes for Covid-related smell problems, but our understanding of these conditions suggests that things will resolve in the majority of cases.

In general, in the first three weeks after developing smell loss, no interventions are necessary. If the smell loss persists beyond three weeks, then it is worth exploring smell training, peer support and other interventions/supplements as discussed below.

FLUCTUATIONS

Many people report that during the recovery period, they experience fluctuations in their recovering sense of smell. This can be very upsetting and can often feel like you've dropped back to square one. It is entirely normal for the Covid recovery process. So don't worry too much, and just remember that every day is just one day. Tomorrow may be better.

Why smell loss can get you down

Scientific studies into how loss of smell affects people's mental health have found that over a longer period, loss of smell leads to feelings of isolation, sadness and depression. You may no longer feel attracted to your partner, or you might not feel you can bond with your baby. These things happen when smell is interrupted, is entirely normal, and you should feel reassured that for the vast majority, all this will improve. Sometimes it is helpful to find time to pause; try to get outside into nature, take care to notice other sensory experiences, such as birdsong or the movement of clouds, and practise relaxation techniques, yoga or meditation.

A GUIDE TO PAROSMIA

We know that parosmia, the term used to describe an alteration in smell perception, can arrive at any time after Covid – sometimes immediately, sometimes many months after the first infection. There are also people who experience parosmia only, with no smell loss.

Parosmia can be very hard to live with. The first few weeks are generally the hardest. Most people report finding certain foods, such as meat, onions, garlic, eggs and coffee, as well as toothpaste and many other common food and household items, triggering the feeling of disgust and sometimes nausea. This creates all kinds of problems for people, especially when living in a family environment or in the workplace where you might be exposed to other people's food smells, perfume or other triggers.

In the worst phases of parosmia, you might feel sick, want to be sick, not feel hungry or not want to eat anything at all. Using a nose clip can be helpful if you are cooking for others or need to be present where food is being consumed. It can also be helpful to use calorie replacement drinks. Ask your doctor about this if you have been struggling with your appetite loss due to parosmia. If you are losing a significant amount of weight, you should seek medical advice.

'It started with a fried egg. I just kept smelling something off and I thought maybe it was a bad egg. I made a fried egg a few days later with a new batch of eggs...and there it was again. The next day I made hard boiled eggs for my husband and there was that smell again. It was the egg white. I literally had to spit it out. And it's been getting worse ever since. My hot water has the same smell. As does coffee. Onions. Chicken. Any kind of beef. Pork. Baby wipes... Fresh rain... I literally add to the list every single day. Every day something else takes on the same god-awful smell.'

There are no medications for parosmia, and there is nothing we know about yet that might make it go away, so it is likely to be a long haul. Here are some tips that will help you manage it, and enable you to get enough calories to keep you going:

Stick to bland and room-temperature foods
Many people say that they can eat things like boiled rice, plain pasta and plain yogurt. Cheese is often safe, too. Foods that are at room temperature or cool give off less smell than hot things, so keep that in mind.

Avoid things that are fried, roasted or grilled
This goes for everything, from chips to roasted peanuts. The roasting process gives off aroma chemicals that we know are very difficult for people with parosmia to deal with. Poached chicken or fish might be OK, but fish and chips might be a 'no' for you.

Keep experimenting
You should keep trying foods in small quantities to find out what is tolerable, and what is not. Keep a list on the fridge, and mark down what is 'safe' and what's a trigger. What you can tolerate may well be different from other people, so keep experimenting. You might try doing this with a partner, as it can be stressful. What's a trigger for parosmia today might have changed in two weeks. Many people have described this. Parosmia can be a constantly changing picture.

'I adapted my diet quite quickly. I replaced meat with lentils and pulses and dairy with plant-based alternatives. I avoided onions and garlic and replaced with chilli and fennel. I found myself appreciating texture a lot more, and focusing on that as a way to get enjoyment out of food. I used the opportunity to try new foods and I'm eating foods now that I never ate before. I'm exploring different ways of cooking and being more creative now my parosmia has eased. I'm really trying to make something good out of it.'

The supermarket and cooking

Food shopping with parosmia can be a demoralising experience. It might be helpful, especially if you still have to cook for family members, to plan menus and order your food online. Try to avoid spending more time than you need to in the supermarket, as the smells can be overwhelming. If you prepare something that you truly can't face eating, just remember that this is common, and many people with parosmia have experienced it. The main thing is to eat something – whatever you feel able to stomach.

Engage your close family and friends to help you on this journey

People with complex health conditions often rely on family members to help them with hospital visits, emotional support and practical matters. In the case of parosmia, this strategy can also be very effective. Because it is an invisible condition, you might be reluctant to 'make a fuss', especially if no one understands. Helping those closest to you to know what is happening is crucial if you are to get the support you need. You might find that sharing this book with your loved ones helps.

Parosmia is a sign that things are healing

The distorted smells of parosmia are recognised by researchers to be an indicator that healing is happening. It's very difficult to live with, but it may make it a bit easier to know that it is a good sign.

What treatments work?

The British Rhinological Society and Ear, Nose and Throat (ENT) UK have created guidelines for doctors on how to advise patients who have experienced smell problems after Covid. Leading doctors were asked to give their opinion on a number of treatments and two courses of action were agreed: smell training, with peer support, and steroid nasal sprays.

You may have heard about the use of certain supplements that have been discussed in the press, such as alpha lipoic acid, omega 3 oils, vitamin A drops for the nose, and zinc. The evidence for these supplements is not yet strong enough, or the research is too preliminary, to recommend them. This does not mean that they are definitely not helpful; some of them are still being studied. If you wish to try these supplements, remember to follow dosage instructions carefully.

Smell training and peer support

The evidence for smell training is now well established. Some simple instructions on smell training follow. Combining smell training with peer support groups is another way for you to share your concerns, your questions, your little successes and your setbacks. This is especially important where often family members or close friends can't relate to your experience. Isolation is a common feeling when you have lost your sense of smell, so joining in groups and sharing those feelings can be so helpful.

Steroid nasal sprays

Steroid nasal sprays can be useful in controlling inflammation, and therefore swelling, inside the nose, and thereby improve the functioning of the olfactory pathway. They are recommended in the guidelines mentioned above after two weeks of smell loss. Some sprays can be bought over the counter, or you can ask your doctor. It's important that you understand exactly how to use your spray bottle. Simple demonstration videos, created together with the British Rhinological Society, are available at AbScent.org/NoseWell.

How to use smell training as a tool for recovery

While you cannot completely control your recovery, there are simple, proven strategies that can help. Having said that, the first lesson here is to be kind to yourself and allow all the time you need to take care of yourself. No one can know what it is like to have your nose, or your appetite.

Self-test

If you are going to start smell training, it can be helpful to try to pinpoint where you are now with your sense of smell. And then you can revisit this test in a few weeks or months and note any progress. How you self-test is up to you. You could make a list of 10–20 things in your kitchen, and smell them, noting any experiences you have. Do you smell anything at all? Just a sort of 'nothing' smell that is meaningless? Is it very distorted and makes you feel nauseous? Make your list, and also note how you feel. Then stick it to the fridge and check in with it occasionally. Try not to do this every day. Like getting on the bathroom scales daily, this isn't really helpful. Once a month is plenty. Once you've self-tested, get yourself ready for smell training.

Smell training: the basics

Smell training, also called olfactory training, is a supportive technique that might help you recover more quickly from your smell loss. This technique has been studied since 2009, and there is sound scientific evidence that it can speed up your recovery. Smell training isn't a cure in the traditional sense, but rather a way to make recovery faster.

Smell training consists of smelling something with a strong odour, like essential oils or spices from your kitchen cupboard, for a couple of minutes twice daily. It is easy to do, but it is important that you understand a little bit about how and why it works. In this section, we will help you make your own kit, and then take you through a smell-training session.

What do I need to do?

It helps to have a kit to do your training with. You can easily make your own:

You will need

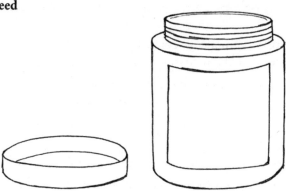

- Small (30ml/1oz) amber glass jars* (essential oils are volatile and will degrade quickly in sunlight – the amber glass protects them). Order online or buy at your local store.
- Blotting paper, watercolour paper or any heavy paper that is white/ uncoloured.
- 4 bottles of essential oils** (there is nothing magical about essential oils – they are just easily obtainable, affordable and strong smelling).
- Adhesive labels to mark the jars and lids.

* You can have as many jars as you like, but make four as a minimum.
** Alternatively, use a few drops of food flavourings such as vanilla, or dry spices.

TIP
Select smells that are familiar to you. It helps to choose smells that are meaningful to you and are tied to more vivid memories and emotions. Examples include citrus fruits or smells associated with Christmas, such as cinnamon and cloves.

Directions
- Cut circles from the paper to fit into the bottom of the jars.
- Add a few drops of each of the oils on to the paper discs.
- Attach labels to the jars and lids, writing the contents and the date on the label.

How to keep the jars fresh
Keep your jars out of sunlight and away from heat. Things that have a strong smell, like essential oils, often lose their character in heat and sunlight. So protect them, and make sure to keep the lids on tightly between uses.

Do I need to top the jars up?
Your kit should be good for four months. You can, of course, top up the jars sooner, but it is probably not necessary.

Why is the kit made the way it is?
After lots of trial and error, and feedback from thousands of people, the jar method has been found to be the best. Why? Because it inspires confidence that you are getting the strongest scent possible when you train. The small amount of air in the jar carrying the scent is available to your nose when you open it.

The amber-coloured glass jars are recommended over clear jam jars because they exclude light and protect the essential oils, keeping them fresh for longer. Blotting paper is recommended over things like cotton wool and kitchen paper, which have loosely packed fibres that can harbour bacteria and cause the smell to go off. Of course, cotton wool is better than nothing, if that is all you have available – just refresh the jars weekly.

The smell-training practice
The most important thing to know about smell training is that it takes time and is a long-term commitment. If you are part of the longer-term smell loss recovery group, you'll need to do it twice a day for a minimum of four months. Like stroke rehabilitation, smell training takes time and concentration – it is work for the brain, not just the nose – so if you only do it a couple of times a week and then stop after a few weeks, you are bound to be disappointed. The best results come from twice daily attention to smell training.

The method
Each individual session should only last 3–5 minutes. Pick a quiet time of the day when you can concentrate and try to find somewhere free from distraction. Turn off music, the television, your computer or anything else that might distract you.

Opening one jar at a time, close your eyes and bring the jar to your nose. Inside the jar will be a concentration of the smell. Try to capture that as you breathe in, taking very small 'bunny sniffs'. By this, we mean drawing in just enough air to go into the nose, rather than all the way down into the lungs. While you are doing this, try to imagine the smell. Can you remember anything in your past that could help you conjure up the smell?

If you can, try to replay this memory. If it is lemon, try to remember something about it, maybe cutting a lemon, or squeezing a lemon. In your mind, try to feel the peel of the lemon on your fingertips, the lemon oil coming up from the pores on the skin of the fruit. Sniff and think. After these short sniffs, you might pause and breathe normally for a few breaths, then go back to the bunny sniffs.

When you've done this for 30 seconds or so, put the lid back on the jar. Again, take some normal breaths. Now do the same with the three other jars.

Now for the important part…
…Thinking about what you are trying to smell.

The most important thing about smell training isn't what you are smelling, but what your brain is doing while you are trying to smell. In other words, you could smell-train with a jar of rubber bands, and it would be just as good, as long as you could picture rubber bands in your mind, or perhaps recall the smell of plimsolls from your time in school. Or maybe it would remind you of the smell of a fresh can of tennis balls. Wherever you go in your smell-training practice, try to recall memories that are as vivid as possible.

The great big takeaway: smell training is about using your mind and memory, not just your nose.

Let's look at some commonly reported problems
I can't smell anything! I must be doing it wrong!
If you've lost your sense of smell, you won't feel anything from the jars at first. In the beginning, it will be a leap of faith for you to do smell training. Concentrate while you do it, keep your mind on remembering smells, and wait and see what happens.

I can't remember any smells! Help!

Some people really struggle to conjure up any smell memories at all. Try this exercise: think of a very happy experience when you were a child, perhaps a holiday. It really helps if the occasion involved food. Now imagine your favourite food from this memory. See it on the plate. Remember the colour and the texture. If you were involved in the cooking, remember the feel of it in your hands. If you were a child then, was it sticky? Hot? Cold? Who served the food? Can you remember who was with you? Take your time in thinking about this – it won't happen instantly. Now revisit the idea of the smell of that food. Can you get close?

Nope. I can't do it. How else can I use my smell memory and brain when smell training?

Don't worry – not everyone is able to remember smells. You can try another technique. This simply involves shutting out all other sensory stimulus – noise, light (close your eyes) – then sitting quietly and sharpening your attention to wait for any 'signal'. Imagine you are looking into a deep well, and you can't see the bottom. You drop a pebble in. The water level might be a very long way down. The more time that goes by without hearing a 'plop', the more you know the sound will be faint. It is this way when you are trying to grasp the very first, faint smell signals. You need to wait, and be observant.

I just can't believe this works – I'm sceptical.

There is clear evidence that smell training can help to facilitate the return of smell. However, it does require persistence and the payoff is slow and sometimes imperceptible. The process requires quite a lot of trust. For some people, especially when they are struggling and having a difficult time with long-term symptoms, this can feel a little bit daunting. But if you think about it as one small thing you have control over, it can feel empowering. This is a simple thing that you can feel you have accomplished every day. A tiny step on a long road. So try to keep going.

Here are some other ways of working the smell-training experience into your day, without even trying.

- Pay attention to the scent of your hand sanitiser or hand cream when you use it.
- Put a drop of essential oil on your bookmark and have a sniff when you sit down to read.
- Use scented lip balm.
- Explore the scent of your body-care products every time you use them.
- Break off a few leaves and crush them when you are out on a walk. Have a good sniff.
- When you hug your partner, linger a bit longer and try to feel their personal smell.
- Put a drop of essential oil on the outside of your face mask. (Make sure you are using a skin-friendly essential oil.)

SUMMARY

- Smell loss is very personal, and no one really knows what it is like except you.

- Try to share as much as you can with family and friends. If this is too challenging, sharing with others in the same position can help.

- It's normal to feel low and isolated when you're experiencing smell loss.

- Your food preferences will change frequently, so keep experimenting.

- Recovery can take a long time, sometimes up to two years. It can be frustrating, but there is hope.

- Smell training is a wonderful way to support yourself. Remember that, like stroke rehabilitation, smell training requires a long-term commitment. We recommend twice daily for a minimum of four months.

- Parosmia is a sign that things are improving.

- Most people will regain some, or all, of their sense of smell in time.

CHAPTER 8

Other Long Covid symptoms

In addition to fatigue, breathlessness and smell impairment, there are many other recognised symptoms in Long Covid, ranging from brain fog and dizziness to hair loss and gastrointestinal upset. This chapter will provide a description of some of the more common of these symptoms and offer advice and management strategies.

Brain fog

Brain fog is a term used by sufferers of Long Covid to describe symptoms related to thinking, memory and attention. Many sufferers describe feeling fuzzy-headed or absent-minded, having problems with their memory, difficulty finding words and heightened sensitivity to sensations such as loud noise or touch. For some, sustaining enough attention to be able to read or watch television becomes difficult. The lengthy and numerous video meetings that have become commonplace during the pandemic can be overwhelming. Socialising, with all its complex cues and attentional demands that may have previously come naturally, becomes wearing.

> 'The name brain fog doesn't do justice to the experience.
> Practically, it means that you can't think right. It turns out that
> thinking is pretty core to meaningful existence! At my worst, over
> several minutes, I couldn't work out a seatbelt.'

Brain fog is associated with other conditions in addition to Long Covid, such as fibromyalgia and ME/CFS. Fatigue, common to all these conditions, can significantly impact on our thinking. Indeed, brain fog and fatigue are intimately connected for many people, and as such, some call brain fog 'cognitive fatigue'.

You may be worried that brain fog is a sign that you're developing dementia. We can reassure you that there is no evidence that infection with Covid-19 causes dementia. Research* has been carried out using tests of cognitive function and found that although those who had had Covid-19 scored lower, particularly around sustained attention, these scores improved over time. This is mirrored in our experience, and we usually see brain fog improving over time, in parallel with other symptoms.

> 'My memory became so bad I was convinced I was developing Alzheimer's. My grandmother lived with Alzheimer's for years so I saw how bad it can get. After Covid, I forgot words, I kept losing my keys and forgetting conversations I'd had. It was petrifying.'

Brain fog can be incredibly frustrating and deeply unsettling. It can impact on your ability and/or confidence to do your job, whether that is at home or in an office. It can affect how you relate to yourself and to those around you.

Strategies

- Many people with Long Covid report that their brain fog is closely related to their fatigue. If you find this is the case, then please do go back and read chapter 2, Managing Fatigue. Strategies of **pacing and energy preservation** may help you to manage your brain fog.
- **Compensatory strategies** such as creating to-do lists or keeping a diary can be helpful. While not a fix for the symptoms, these strategies can help reduce the impact brain fog has on your daily life.
- It can be helpful to examine whether your brain fog follows a **pattern** or has predictable fluctuations.
- Aim to **organise your day and plan tasks** to take advantage of any times that you regularly feel more mental clarity.
- Try to **avoid triggers**. For example, some people find that drinking alcohol or being inactive worsens their brain fog.
- If your other symptoms allow it, **light exercise** can improve brain fog.
- **Improving your sleep** can be helpful as well. Chapter 4 contains practical strategies on how to do this.

---

* Zhao, S. et al (2022) 'Rapid vigilance and episodic memory decrements in COVID-19 survivors.' *Brain Communications*, 4(1). https://doi.org/10.1093/braincomms/fcab295

- **Stress, low mood and anxiety** can have a big impact on our thinking and processing. Addressing these may help improve your brain fog.
- It is also important to remember that it is very human to make mistakes, forget words and 'lose the thread'. Worry about brain fog can make the symptoms worse. **Practising acceptance** of the brain fog may in fact help.
- Our thinking skills lose 'fitness' quickly if not used. This might be the case for you if you have been away from your usual activities or work for some time. As you slowly **reintroduce your usual activities**, you might find your mental sharpness improves.

Dizziness, vertigo and imbalance

Many people with Long Covid struggle with dizziness. Even before the Covid-19 pandemic, it was known that viruses can sometimes cause persisting dizziness. Although not dangerous, dizziness can be extremely unpleasant and difficult to manage.

Some people develop dizziness and balance problems during or after their initial Covid-19 illness. Others may have had these problems before they got Covid-19 and find their symptoms have worsened afterwards. Symptoms normally improve as you recover over weeks and months, but some people can experience dizziness, vertigo and imbalance for a long time afterwards.

We don't yet fully understand how Covid-19 affects our balance systems. However, we have come to recognise that some of the strategies our bodies use to get through the initial infection can start to drive the dizziness once the acute illness itself settles. In effect, our body adapts to the presence of a virus and does not reset naturally once the virus is no longer present.

How balance works

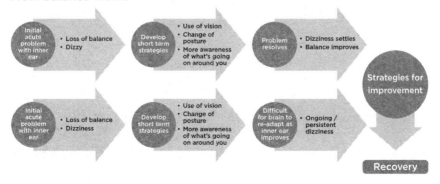

The chart on p. 137 shows different pathways of recovery after an episode of dizziness and this can happen over different lengths of time for different people.

> *'I felt like I was constantly on a ship during a storm. Whenever I moved, I felt like I was about to fall over. If I leaned forward, the whole room would spin. I was completely incapacitated.'*

Our balance system is complicated. Think what your body would need to remain stable while traversing a narrow bridge. It requires information from your vestibular (balance) system, the body position sensors in your joints, and muscles and skin to stay upright. You sense where you are in space through seeing objects around you, feeling the movement of your head, the position of your joints, and the muscle tension in your upper body, arms, back, stomach, buttocks and legs.

We can sometimes rely too much on our vision. When we do this, balance, vertigo and fatigue can become worse. It can also contribute to the feeling of brain fog. This information helps us to understand how to start to address dizziness through rehabilitation strategies.

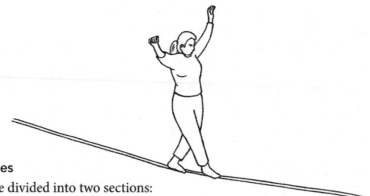

Strategies

These are divided into two sections:

1. Managing acute dizziness.
2. Managing persistent dizziness.

Managing acute dizziness

- Start by thinking about and **planning your everyday activities**.
- You may find getting out of bed will be a challenge. **Sit on the edge of the bed for a minute or two and wait for the dizziness to pass** before

trying to stand. Initially it may be necessary to ask someone to be with you when you try to stand up and walk around.

- Aim to **move normally**. Movement involving your eyes, head and body has been shown to help reduce dizziness and improve balance and fatigue in some conditions affecting the balance system.
- **Be safe.** Plan activities to improve your balance. For example, practise balance in a corner, by a work surface, next to your bed or in a doorway etc. and have someone with you if needed. Do it at a time in the day that suits your body and mind and monitor exertion and recovery levels.
- **Be kind to yourself.** Have a 'setback plan' – for example, evaluate what contributed to the setback, prioritise some activities, have rest periods and plan easy short-term activity goals.
- **Monitor symptoms** and modify your plan as needed.
- Remember the three Ps of fatigue management; **prioritise, plan and pace.**
- When starting or progressing activities, **consider post-exertional malaise** (PEM), recovery times and fatigue.
- Stay within **comfortable ranges of movement** and activity.
- You may feel mildly dizzy during movement. Reassure yourself **it's OK to feel mild dizziness** and you are safe. Dizziness should stop within 1–2 minutes of being still.
- Try to **actively look around**, moving your head to look at different objects while sitting or walking around. Move your head gently at first and slowly increase the directions and speed as you feel able.
- **Try not to be too focused on dizziness** when you are practising. This stops your automatic body movement occurring and can lead to more fatigue. **Try to focus on something else** at the same time because targeting your vision while moving will help your brain adjust more quickly. For example, when you are walking and moving your head, see if you can spot green objects, read road signs or be nosy and watch people. Whatever you prefer to target your vision on! This will allow you to turn your head more automatically without your brain's 'spotlight' being on the dizziness or movement.
- **Target your vision** to pick out details of things near and far away in all directions. For example, as you walk, look at pictures on the wall or patterns on the wallpaper, or, if outside, tree bark, leaves or flowers.

Try to pick out everything that is a specific colour on your route. Move your head more and practise looking side to side, targeting your vision as if you are crossing a road. First go gently and gradually increase the speed of the head turns over time, within your controlled limits.

- **Track birds in the sky**, the movement of animals, raindrops on the window, or watch a ball as you throw and catch it. Remember details and compare them the next time you see them on your walk.
- **Use your hearing aids or glasses** for everyday activities if you have/ need them. This is shown to improve postural stability and balance.

Managing persistent dizziness

Balance rehabilitation exercises can help retrain your balance, reduce dizziness and improve strength, especially if your balance centre is under-working. You can start with the movements below and modify speed and number of repetitions and do less or more movements as your tolerance allows. Aim to do the activities below 1–3 times a day for a total time of at least 12 minutes daily in the acute phase, if tolerance and fatigue allow. You can build this up to 20 minutes spread through the day if you are able.

- **Turn your head to look from side to side.** Try to target your vision on objects near and far, left to right. When comfortable, increase gradually as your recovery time and symptoms allow.
- **Move your head to look up to the ceiling and then look down**, taking your chin to your chest. Try to target your vision by looking at something on the ceiling and floor. When comfortable, increase gradually as your recovery time and symptoms allow.

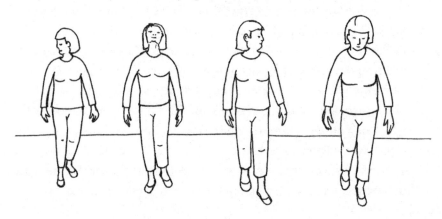

- Sitting down, **bend forwards to take your head and shoulders towards your lap, then return upright**. Alternatively, on standing, bend at the hips to take your head and shoulders forwards and down, reaching with your hands towards a chair seat, then return to an upright position. When comfortable, increase gradually as your recovery time and symptoms allow.

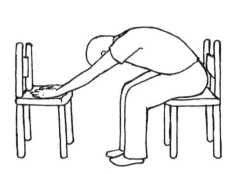 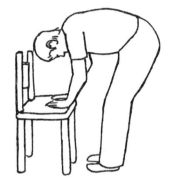

- **Practise closing your eyes while sitting or standing still with your feet apart.** Begin by focusing on the weight distributed through your feet.
- While sitting or standing, **wiggle or squeeze your toes and pay attention to the sensation of the ground beneath your feet.** Close your eyes for 10 seconds. Increase gradually as you become steadier and more confident. You may feel a gentle sway and this is normal. Try to keep the weight evenly distributed over your feet. Progress to standing with your feet together.
- **Practise standing with your feet apart and sway side to side** or rotate right and left, letting your arms hang loosely, with your eyes open or closed and within your tolerance and safety limits.
- **Practise standing up and sitting down with your eyes open** to start with and progress to doing it with your eyes closed, without using your hands if possible. Do this in a safe place – for example, at a table or from your bed. Repeat as able. Build up your tolerance gradually and monitor dizziness and fatigue. It is normal to feel strange and a little dizzy or disorientated with your eyes closed.
- **While standing, look at a target and move your head halfway from side to side** (turn) without losing clear sight of the target (as if you are

shaking your head to say 'no, no, no'). Repeat for 10 seconds or until you feel (1–3 out of 10) dizzy. Do this 1–3 times daily.

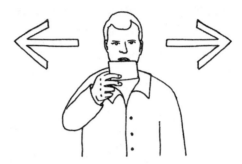

- **While standing, look at a target and move your head halfway up and down** (nod) without losing clear sight of the target. Repeat for 10 seconds or until you feel (1–3 out of 10) dizzy. Do this 1–3 times daily. Any dizziness triggered by these movements should settle in 1–2 minutes. Modify the movements by increasing or decreasing the time or repetitions you do them for as required. Do 7 days at the same level before increasing the time or repetitions in small, gradual stages.

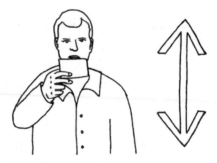

A health professional specially trained in vestibular and balance rehabilitation (usually a specialist vestibular/balance physiotherapist or audiologist) can help if symptoms persist.

> If you continue to experience these symptoms or if they worsen, it is important to contact your healthcare provider as further investigations may be appropriate

SUMMARY

- Dizziness is a recognised complication following viral infections, including Covid-19.

- Although understandable, avoiding movement due to dizziness can slow down your recovery.

- Movement and activity can help reduce dizziness but should be done at the right level for you.

- Symptoms of dizziness generally improve over time and the exercises given here can assist in the recovery process.

Pain

Pain is a common and sometimes under-recognised symptom of Long Covid. If you experience any new pains, then please consult with your healthcare provider as a first step.

People with Long Covid commonly experience persisting generalised muscle pains. For some, the pains are similar to those experienced during their acute Covid-19 illness or during flu. There may be associated joint pains or pains in the bones. The pains follow different patterns in different individuals but many find that the pains move around, affecting different muscle groups over time. Some find that the pains are relieved by movement, others feel that movement makes the pain worse. Some people notice that the pains are worse in the morning, others experience worse pain at night.

Pain is one way that the body keeps us safe from potential harm. Acute pain is often a signal from the body that there is an infection, an injury or inflammation. However, the link between persistent pain and bodily damage is less clear. In persistent pain, the pain signalling pathways themselves become sensitised and begin to fire automatically. A misfiring pain pathway will signal to the brain that there is a potentially harmful stimulus when in fact there is no actual damage or danger. Unfortunately, we are not able to distinguish between pain that is caused by damage to our bodies and pain that is caused by misfiring of the pain pathways themselves. Both are real and distressing.

'Pain. Everywhere. In joints, in muscles, in tendons, in my head. Everywhere. And nothing helped it. It's like all the deepest tissues had been stretched out on a rock and whacked with a hammer. The pain in my back and chest was insane and still troubles me today.'

Everyone experiences and responds to pain differently. Pain can trigger the 'fight or flight' response, leading to a rapid heart rate and increased blood pressure. This is an important and natural bodily response that enables you to protect yourself in the face of potential harm. However, in the context of persistent pain when there is no actual bodily threat, this response itself can become a problem, driving our anxiety and distress.

Pain is deeply unpleasant. In order to try to ease it, we often avoid doing what we think might trigger or worsen it, such as moving. Unfortunately, reducing movement can result in our muscles weakening or stiffening and can worsen the pain further.

Pain can be challenging to manage. We have listed below practical strategies that our patients have found helpful. Some of these strategies are aimed at directly reducing the pain itself. Others are focused on improving quality of life in the context of pain.

Strategies

- If you have reached a point where pain has limited your ability to live your life the way you used to, it is useful to start upon your path of recovery by **setting yourself small, achievable goals**. These might include getting out of bed at a certain time each day, or increasing the distance you walk by 20 metres every week.
- **Record your goals** and whether you are achieving them. It is important for you to document and see your progress, even if it is very slow. You may not achieve all your goals, and that is completely OK.
- Try to **move daily**. Understand that pain-free movement may not be possible at first, so keep it limited. Any movement should be paced and care taken to avoid exacerbating your fatigue or triggering any post-exertional malaise. Please refer to chapter 5 for clear guidance on reintroducing exercise.
- Try to identify what activities make you feel good, your '**nourishing activities**', and build these into your daily routine. For example, some

people find that practising mindfulness meditation can make them feel overall better, so they might try to schedule a 10-minute meditation each morning or evening.

- Also try to identify and avoid **unhelpful protective behaviours**. These might include being sedentary or drinking more alcohol, for example.
- Finding a way to **improve sleep** can be helpful (*see* chapter 4).
- **Gentle massage,** carried out by yourself, a loved one or a professional, can help to retrain the misfiring pain signal pathway and ease your pain.
- **Acupuncture** is recommended in the treatment of some forms of persistent pain and may be helpful in Long Covid.
- Speak to and **share your experience and your goals** with your family and loved ones. This can help them to be your cheerleaders on your recovery journey.

SENSORY CHANGES

Changes in sensation experienced by people with Long Covid include tingling and numbness in fingers or on patches of skin. Other commonly reported symptoms include burning sensations on the chest or arms. These sensory changes often seem to move and change over time – for example, on some days they affect the legs and on others the arms.

> 'Then [I had] some weird symptoms. For six months, my eyesight got progressively worse; then, it got better. A dull ache halfway up my left arm, always happening at exactly the same time as a sharp stabbing pain in my Adam's apple.'

Some people with Long Covid report all-over body tingling, or experience an intermittent electric shock-like sensation or hypersensitivity of their skin. These sensory changes appear to be driven by similar changes in the nervous system that drive persistent pain. As such, the same management strategies apply here.

Palpitations

The term 'palpitations' is used to describe the sensation of an awareness of your own heart beating. Over half of patients with Long Covid report palpitations and/or a fast heartbeat. Serious cardiac problems, however, do not appear to be any more common in Long Covid than they are in the general population. Most healthy people experience palpitations at least occasionally, often triggered by factors such as stress or anxiety. Palpitations can last from a few seconds to many hours. Most people are aware of their heart beating when anxious or stressed, such as before a job interview or when exercising. This is a normal bodily response.

Ectopic beats are early (premature) or extra heartbeats. They can be thought of as 'hiccups' and often lead to a short pause or slowing of the heart after them. They are often experienced as a 'missed' beat. Ectopic beats are found in almost everyone, although some people notice them more than others. They are usually harmless and don't need treatment unless they occur very often or cause severe symptoms.

In most cases, palpitations are not serious. They can, however, be a nuisance. Palpitations that are associated with blackouts, severe dizziness or chest pain may need urgent attention, however, and should be reported promptly to your doctor.

We have observed that the most common finding in people with Long Covid is a disproportionately high heart rate in response to physical activity. Many people find that their heart rate rises rapidly on even minimal exertion (for example, just walking across a room or preparing a meal).

This phenomenon has also been recognised by cardiologists following other viral infections, long before Covid appeared. It is known as inappropriate sinus tachycardia (IST) – 'sinus' means 'normal heart rhythm' and 'tachycardia' means 'fast heart rate'. So, this is just the normal faster heart rate that we all experience when we need our heart rate to go faster – for example, when we exercise – but it is happening when it shouldn't be, or too vigorously, so it is referred to as 'inappropriate'. A network of nerves in the body, known as the autonomic nervous system, controls many of the automatic bodily functions, such as our heart rate, blood pressure, breathing and digestion. Covid appears to somehow increase the sensitivity of these nerves, driving some of the symptoms commonly experienced, including the fast heart rate.

These fast heart rate episodes do not damage the heart, do not increase risk of heart attacks, and do not increase risk of stroke, however unpleasant the symptoms may be. Although it can take some time to settle down, over time (sometimes many months or even longer), it usually will. This has been found to be the case for many people with the same problem after other viral illnesses.

Sometimes, the natural changes in the heartbeat when you stand up can be exaggerated and this can lead to symptoms. For example, the heart rate should rise a few beats when we stand up. However, an abnormally high and sustained rise in the heart rate on standing can occur (again, probably due to an effect on the autonomic nervous system). This is characteristic of what is referred to as postural orthostatic tachycardia syndrome (PoTS). It can also be associated with dizziness and fainting.

In PoTS, there is an abnormally large increase in the heart rate after sitting up or standing. In addition to palpitations, symptoms can include dizziness or feeling light-headed, and fatigue. Like inappropriate sinus tachycardia, it is not in any way life threatening and will normally get better with time, but can be very unpleasant.

For both inappropriate sinus tachycardia and PoTS, simple, practical self-management strategies can help to relieve your symptoms.

Strategies

- **Move slowly between lying and upright positions**, and avoid long periods of standing.
- **Stay well hydrated** through the day. Aim for 2–3 litres of non-caffeinated, non-alcoholic fluid each day.
- Having **small and frequent meals**, rather than three large meals, appears to be better tolerated and can ease PoTS symptoms.
- **Try simple manoeuvres before and on standing:** move your arms and legs before you stand and squeeze your buttocks 5–10 times on standing.
- **Wait until the dizziness has settled before walking.**
- Try to **establish a balanced diet** of protein, vegetables, dairy and fruit.
- **Have a big drink of water before moving.**
- **Increase your salt intake.** Many people find that increasing the amount of salt in their diet can help with these symptoms. High-salt-containing foods include stock cubes, anchovies, crisps and cheese.
- **Avoid hot environments.**

MEDICATIONS FOR A RAPID HEART RATE

The strategies listed above need time to take effect. If, after a few months, your symptoms remain troubling, your doctor may consider prescribing a medication such as a beta blocker to try to control your heart rate. However, it is worth noting that medications are not always effective and can come with side effects. Some people will find these worse than the rapid heart rate itself.

Most importantly, remember that an inappropriately fast heart rate ('inappropriate sinus tachycardia') will not cause your body harm.

Chest pain

There are many reasons people develop pains and discomfort in the chest area. These symptoms are common following viral infections, including Covid-19 – indeed, chest pain is one of the most frequently reported symptoms in Long Covid. Most chest pain is not a sign of anything serious, but see your doctor if you have started experiencing new chest pain. In many cases, your doctor can be confident that there is not a serious cause for the pain by listening carefully to your description of the symptoms. In some cases, additional tests may be needed.

There has been concern raised regarding the possibility of inflammation of the heart, known as myocarditis. This is something that can occur with any viral illness but is rarely of any clinical significance. Once your doctor is happy that he or she has ruled out a serious cause, the focus can turn to understanding and dealing with your symptoms.

> 'Chest pain and compression for 12 months that made it feel like I was trapped under the wheel of a car. The pain was agonising and radiated down my left arm. I could have called 999 every day for a year. I did once, and all tests were clear.'

Although your doctor can confidently rule out a serious cause for chest pain, it is sometimes more difficult to know exactly what the cause is. Many organs lie near or within the chest. These include the heart, lungs, lung walls, muscles, ribs, blood vessels, nerves, stomach and oesophagus, among others. Pain can arise from any of these structures. However, for many people with Long Covid, the exact origin of the chest pain is not clear. Medical investigations are almost universally normal and virtually all chest pain we see is non-threatening. The key is to find a way of managing the pain. Chest pain can be a source of worry, even if your doctor has ruled out serious causes. Fortunately, there are some helpful strategies that can help relieve the pain.

Strategies

- Although it was once recommended that people with chest pains arising from chest wall muscles and joints kept very still, we suggest that people with chest pains and Long Covid make a **gradual return to their usual activities**, including gentle stretching, exercise and breathing exercises.
- If there is a specific point of the chest that is causing discomfort, **hot or cold packs** can be helpful.
- Some people find that **painkillers**, including paracetamol and anti-inflammatories, can be helpful.

Headaches

Some people with Long Covid experience troubling and often persistent headaches. Some describe headaches that are felt diffusely over the neck, scalp and forehead. Others report a pain in the back of their neck that travels over their head to their forehead or eyes. The pain can be dull and heavy, or sharp. It can be made worse by stress, fatigue or dehydration. Some find that certain neck movements and changes in posture can worsen the pain.

We commonly reach for the nearest painkiller when we have a headache. This is not, however, always the right thing to do. In some cases, regular daily use of painkillers can itself drive a headache. Doctors sometimes call this 'medication overuse headache'. How painkillers cause headaches in this way is not well understood. The headaches usually settle down when the painkiller is stopped, but this may take time, sometimes weeks to months.

Strategies

- It is important to try to identify the triggers of your headache, if there are any. This can be achieved by starting a **'headache diary'**. Take a few moments when your headache flares to note down what might have triggered it, such as strong emotions, missed meals, poor sleep, fatigue, menstrual hormone changes, over-exertion. Often there is more than one trigger for headache.
- **Pacing**, although mentioned frequently elsewhere in the book, is useful here too. Try to pace out your activities to avoid reaching your headache threshold.
- General **'healthy living'** can make a difference; avoid sleeping too little, use stress management and relaxation techniques, avoid skipping meals, drink plenty of fluids.
- If you do think you might have a medication overuse headache, then consider **weaning off your painkillers** and giving yourself at least one month off to see if the headaches settle.

Tinnitus

'Howling screeching whining tinnitus in both ears every day for 20 months. Like a personal dial-up modem. When I wake up and when I fall asleep. I try and ignore it but some days it drives me mad.'

Tinnitus is an awareness of sound in the ears or head that is not coming from an external source. It appears to be a relatively common symptom experienced by people suffering from Long Covid. There are various different sounds that people describe hearing, including buzzing, ringing or whizzing. Tinnitus may or may not be associated with loss of hearing. In the first instance, it is worth consulting your healthcare provider. While no medications have been proven to treat tinnitus, there are strategies you can try to help manage it.

Strategies

- **Relaxation techniques** can be extremely useful to reduce tinnitus. Many people find that their tinnitus worsens when they are stressed or anxious.

- **Avoid loud noises** and sound – some people choose to wear ear plugs if they need to be in loud environments.
- Even **light exercise,** such as tai chi, has been shown to be effective at reducing tinnitus.
- **Distraction techniques** can be a practical way of managing this condition – some people find their tinnitus reduces when they focus their concentration on something else, such as a task or another sound.
- **White noise** can be helpful to manage tinnitus experienced at night. For example, leaving a fan on or playing soothing background noise, such as jungle or beach sounds.

Gastrointestinal disturbance

'Relentless stomach pain, cramps, nausea, reflux. For 14 months. Nothing brought any relief. Every item of food I consumed just aggravated it.'

Some people with Long Covid experience gastrointestinal disturbance. Most commonly, this is in the form of bloating, a change in bowel habit and abdominal discomfort. If you have experienced a noticeable change in your bowel habit, it is recommended that you see your doctor. You may undergo testing to check that you do not have a condition such as coeliac disease or inflammatory bowel disorder. In Long Covid, it may be that these standard investigations do not reveal another condition. If that is the case, practical management strategies can be helpful.

Strategies
- Try to **reflect on your symptoms** and whether there are any triggers or ways that seem to relieve them. For many Long Covid sufferers, these symptoms flare up in relation to worsening fatigue, so focusing on fatigue management should be a priority (*see* chapter 2).
- **Modify fibre** in your diet. For example, if you tend to have a lot of loose stools, then lowering the fibre in your diet can be helpful. If you have a lot of hard stools, then increasing the fibre can help.
- Remember to **keep yourself well hydrated**.
- Alcohol can make bowel symptoms worse. If you find this is the case,

then try to **reduce your overall alcohol intake** – try to drink no more than 14 units a week.

- **Fatty and processed foods** such as crisps, fried foods and cakes can all aggravate gastrointestinal symptoms. You may find you feel better when these are avoided or reduced.
- **Sweeteners** can cause diarrhoea, so it might be worth trying to avoid these.
- **Stress management and relaxation techniques** can be effective to manage these symptoms.
- To manage bloating, try to **eat small, regular meals**. Oats can also be helpful to ease bloating.
- There is no clear evidence on the use of **probiotics**, but some people with Long Covid have found that their gastrointestinal symptoms improve on them. If you are going to try them, use them for at least a month.
- There are medications that can be used to manage gastrointestinal symptoms, such as antispasmodics, laxatives or anti-motility drugs, but please consult your healthcare practitioner before trialling these.

Hair, nail and skin changes

Some people with Long Covid experience changes in their hair, nails and skin. It is known that various general health conditions affect the hair, nails and skin so it is important to discuss any new symptoms with your doctor and avoid self-diagnosis. Below are some of the more common phenomena that can occur in Long Covid.

Hair loss

Many people suffering from Long Covid experience hair loss or thinning. A scalp condition called telogen effluvium can occur as a result of long-term or acute illness and this may well explain the hair loss seen in Long Covid sufferers. We normally shed around 30 to 150 hairs a day as part of the 'telogen', or shedding phase, of our 'hair cycle'. In telogen effluvium, more of our hair enters the telogen phase and so we start to shed noticeably more hair than normal. You may notice more hair in your shower or bath plughole, or in the hairbrush or comb. The condition does not usually require treatment, and the hair normally grows back after around six months.

Nail changes

Nail growth can be interrupted by ill health. Some Long Covid sufferers develop deep grooves that run side to side in their nails. These are known as 'Beau's lines' and, while not specific to Long Covid, can cause some concern when they appear seemingly out of the blue. There are a number of different causes, but in particular they are seen after acute illness or trauma. Interestingly, it is possible to estimate the date of the triggering event by measuring how far from the nail bed the Beau's line is: fingernails are known to grow at a rate of 0.1mm per day and toenails at a rate of 0.05mm per day.

Rashes

Some people with Long Covid experience generalised skin itchiness without a visible rash. The cause for this is not understood. Itching can be a side effect of medications or be caused by allergic reactions, dermatitis, eczema or some general medical conditions. Sometimes stress can make itching worse. It is worth speaking with your doctor about new skin conditions or rashes. In general, itching can be eased by:

- cool or warm baths;
- contact with a cool or warm wet towel;
- emollient creams;
- wearing loose cotton clothing;
- using fragrance-free soaps;
- relaxation techniques.

SUMMARY

- Long Covid is often more than just fatigue and breathlessness.

- Although the other common symptoms can be severely disabling, cardiac, neurological or gastrointestinal organ damage is extremely rare.

- Practical management strategies have been shown to relieve a broad range of symptoms, including brain fog, gastrointestinal upset, persisting pain, dizziness and palpitations.

- Paradoxically, fear and avoidance of movement can themselves limit improvement in pain and dizziness.

- Recovery from Long Covid is often slow and new symptoms and challenges may occur along the way. Slow and steady wins the race.

CHAPTER 9

Return to Work

In this chapter we discuss the importance of work, the process of returning to your current job (that is, getting ready for work, going back to work and staying in work), support that may be available to you on your return to work and a few resources to help you along the way.

The impact of Covid-19 on the world of work

The pandemic has been hard on both employees and employers. It has seen businesses and organisations having to change rapidly the way that they operate; having to set people up to work safely and effectively at home or in the workplace, managing a constant flow of staff sickness or staff needing to isolate, and for some, needing to close for long periods of time, putting staff on furlough.

One of the things that is most evident is that everyone's work situation has changed. Some changes will be temporary, others more permanent. Some changes may be negative but some positive. If you have had time off work due to ill health, your job and the way you worked pre-pandemic may have changed.

What does work mean to you?

Work of all kinds (whether full-time or part-time, paid or unpaid) is a key part of life for most of us. The reasons we work and value work are individual to each of us. Look at the list below and consider what are the important factors for you personally.

- Financial security
- Structure and routine

- A sense of who you are
- A sense of belonging
- A feeling of value
- A sense of achievement
- Positive mental health
- A career pathway
- Social contact and friendships

By considering this question and understanding the values you hold in relation to work, you can explore what aspects of returning to work are important. This will help to guide you towards the best plan for you.

There is not a universal blueprint for a successful return to work. Everybody is different, every job is different and where you are in your recovery will be different, so there will be a need to explore and consider carefully what will work for you.

Things to consider

You may have lots of questions about returning to work, for example:

- When is it the right time to go back to work?
- Is it safe to return to work?
- How will returning to work affect my sick pay/benefits?
- Will my job still be there?
- Can I do my job now?
- Who can help me get back to work?
- How long might it take?
- What happens if I have a recurrence of symptoms or catch Covid again?
- What if everything has changed at work?
- Should I look for another job?

We may not be able to answer all these questions in this chapter, but we can certainly address some, and give you points to reflect on and guide you to people, places or information that can offer further advice.

A WORD ABOUT FINANCES

- In the UK, while off sick you may be receiving occupational sick pay. Your employer will be able to tell you how much this is and how long it will last.
- If you do not get occupational sick pay, you may be receiving statutory sick pay (SSP), which currently lasts for 28 weeks.
- At the end of SSP, if you are still not fit to return to work, you can apply for Employment Support Allowance (ESA) under Universal Credit.
- There may be other benefits you can apply for. Seek advice from local or national benefit advice services or the Citizens Advice Bureau.
- Your employer may have employee health insurance with varying benefits. If this is the case, you can ask your employer what these are.
- You may have taken out personal health insurance policies that you can draw on while you are off sick. Contact your insurance company to find out the details.

When is the right time to be going back to work?

It is natural to want to return to work and to feel that when you do, life will be getting back to normal, especially when you may have been away from work for a long time. However, it is important not to go back too soon or too quickly. Rushing back can result in you feeling that your symptoms are getting worse. This can lead to further time off work and loss of confidence – making you more anxious about trying again.

Remember, from the information around pacing in chapter 2, Managing Fatigue, it is 'slow and steady' that wins the race.

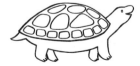 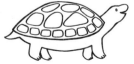 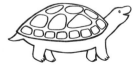

While it is important not to go back too soon, conversely, avoiding going back to work for too long may knock your confidence and as a result make it seem a bigger hurdle to negotiate.

Returning to work is usually a key part of your recovery. Waiting until you are fully recovered before contemplating going back may mean you could be waiting a long time. However, it may be worth remembering that it will likely be in a different way to how it was before. It might involve a phased return, shorter hours, a different environment or perhaps undertaking different duties, at least for a while. We will explore these aspects in more detail further on in the chapter.

Before making any decisions about returning to work, talk things through with people who know you well and who you can trust. This might be your family, colleagues, health professionals and your employer.

Who may be involved in helping you get back to work and what can they do?

Depending on your job and how you are recovering, there are various people who can potentially be involved in supporting you to get back to work. Speak to them to find out what help they can provide. This may include:

AT HOME	
You	• Remember, you are at the centre of your return-to-work journey • It is important that you are involved in all related decisions • You will need to be proactive and take the initiative
Your family and friends	• Can provide general support and advice • Help to problem-solve symptom management and return to work • Accompany you to meetings with your employer, if agreed • Give you practical help getting to and from work if this is difficult • Help you in managing home chores to support you in your return to work

HEALTHCARE PROFESSIONALS	
Long Covid specialist	• Offer advice and recommendations about managing ongoing symptoms and potential implications around return to work • Provide clinic letters that you can share with your employer with recommendations about return to work • Make referrals for further investigations • Refer to specialist therapists for further support, advice and intervention
Primary care physician	• General and specific health advice • Referral for investigations, specialist opinion or therapy • During the time you are considered unfit for work, your primary care physician will provide a Statement of Fitness to Work, usually referred to as a 'fit note' (previously referred to as a 'sick note'). This reports whether you are considered to be (1) not fit for work or (2) fit for work, taking into account any advice provided. (This can draw on information and recommendations from your consultant and/or other healthcare professionals.)
Other health professionals, e.g: • Occupational therapist • Physiotherapist • Psychological services • Speech and language therapist • Dietitian	• Support with ongoing treatment/symptom management • Explore strategies to manage your symptoms • Discuss your readiness and the practicalities around return to work • Provide a letter about what will help you return to work successfully or an Allied Health Professions Health and Work Report about your support needs, supplementing the GP fit note with more detailed recommendations • With your consent – contact your employer to talk about the effects of Long Covid and what would help you to return to work • Where appropriate and practical, speak or meet with you and your employer to agree a return-to-work plan

AT WORK	
Manager and/or HR	• Keep in touch with you while you are off sick • Keep you up to date about work • Give advice, access to policies and procedures • Arrange return-to-work meetings • Work with you to agree a return-to-work plan • Support you once you are back at work • Refer you for additional counselling, therapy and support that may be provided through your workplace
Occupational health (in-house or contracted in)	• Assess readiness to return to work and make recommendations about what adjustments and support you might need
Union representative	• Offer advice and support around work • Accompany and represent you at formal meetings at work
Work colleagues	• Informal contact and support

Steps for getting back to work

Returning to work following a significant illness can be an intricate process and it is usually best to approach this in a structured way – step by step, to reduce the risk of complications. The path to returning to work may not always be smooth and can involve some unexpected setbacks along the way, which take time to overcome before moving forward again. This can be frustrating, but often occurs. If so, some problem-solving with others, such as your partner, family, friends or therapist, may be needed.

It usually helps to break down the process into small, achievable steps towards the overall goal of return to work.

WORD OF CAUTION

The original plan may need to be tweaked several times in response to how it works out in practice. For example, you may find that your return to work takes longer than you had initially thought because you need to consolidate progress before taking further steps. Try to adopt a flexible approach without rigid targets.

When you are making a return-to-work plan, it is often useful to ask yourself some questions to clarify what needs to be included across the overlapping stages: getting ready for work, going back to work, and staying in work, which includes looking after your health at work.

STEP 1: Getting ready for work

Focus on your recovery and rehabilitation

Fatigue, pain and/or breathlessness may be features of Long Covid that you experience. Previous chapters have addressed many strategies and techniques that you can implement to help begin your preparation for returning to work. As part of this, it may help to consider how you can:

- slowly build up structure and routine into your day;
- slowly increase your level of activity/stamina;
- make symptom management an automatic part of your daily routine;
- develop strategies to get around any difficulties (for example, breaking down activities into manageable parts, making to-do lists and reminders, planning and working steadily – rather than rushing through – daily activities, building in regular breaks).

Keep in touch with your employer

Your manager or HR contact may have kept in touch with you to see how you are, whether they can help in any way and also to ask for your current fit note. (Up-to-date guidance on the fit note for patients and employees is detailed on the government website: www.gov.uk/government/publications/the-fit-note-a-guide-for-patients-and-employees/the-fit-note-guidance-for-patients-and-employees)

While you continue to be off work, it is usually helpful to talk to your employer about the best way for them to keep in contact and the frequency of contact. You might prefer a telephone call or contact by email initially, or video conferencing (for example, Zoom, Microsoft Teams).

If there has been no contact from work, you can make contact yourself to keep them up to date with your progress. Contact with your employer will likely increase as you get closer to returning to work.

EMPLOYERS AND COVID-19
Your employer may be having to make many changes because of the pandemic, including reviewing their processes related to return to work to accommodate the effects of Covid-19. As a result, they may be very willing to help but may be under pressure, not know how best to help and look to you and your healthcare professionals to help them to understand your needs.

Consider timings

The right time to go back to work will be different for everyone and there are lots of things to think about. In the first instance, it might be helpful to think about:

- where you are in your recovery;
- the nature of your job – some jobs may be easier to go back to in a gradual way, others are less so;
- other demands – such as financial worries, which may be creating a pressure to return to work sooner than you are ready to;
- whether, having spent time away from work, you wish to rethink priorities in your life (for example, spending more time with your family).

If you are concerned that you will struggle with your old job or you are not sure you wish to return, then you might want to try something different. However, it is important to take time to review your job and support needs and it may not be sensible to rush into any decisions to change your job at this stage.

Reviewing your job

It can help to review the job tasks you do in your role. You could use your job description to help with this (you can ask your employer for this if you do not have one), or make a list of the key tasks that you are involved in.

Think about aspects of your job you feel you could do now and those that may be difficult because of ongoing symptoms. An example of a structured way of reviewing your job through 10 key questions can be found in appendix 1. You could then make a note of any strategies that you think you or your employer could put in place to support you. Below is an example of a structured way of thinking about possible strategies.

Works tasks and potential strategies

Key job tasks	Impact of ongoing symptoms on work	Potential strategies to support work
Getting to internal and external meetings	Takes longer to get there	• Prioritising/clustering meetings • Delegating some meetings to others • Attending some meetings virtually
	Need time to recover from effects of breathlessness	• Build in recovery time prior to meeting
	Build-up of fatigue	• Fatigue management strategies (e.g. pacing/additional short breaks)
Preparing written reports	Distractibility and having lapses in concentration	• Breaking tasks down into smaller parts • Doing demanding tasks when fresh • Using noise-cancelling headphones
	Forgetting key information	• Using memory aids • Recording discussions/meetings
	Fatigue	• Altering work hours • Taking additional short breaks

Start practising elements of your job

It may help to practise work-related skills at home. For example, you could set yourself up with a project that will use your work skills, such as practical work (for example, a DIY project), an administrative task (for example, financial or planning task) or maybe some voluntary work (for example, a support role). This is known as 'work hardening'.

You could speak to your manager to see if there is project work you can do at home to try things out or consider if there is some online training through which you could practise your skills, test yourself out, try out coping strategies and prepare for your return to work.

STEP 2: Going back to work

Those first conversations

When you are preparing to return to work, it is important to have a shared understanding of your difficulties at this time, what helps and what does not. In preparing for discussions about return to work with your employer or for occupational health appointments, it may be helpful to consider and to discuss with someone who knows you well the following questions:

- What is going well, what has improved?
- What is still difficult, what is still an issue, what is not yet back to 100 per cent?
- How does this/would this impact on my work tasks/work role?
- Are there other questions or concerns I want to bring up at the meeting?

Discuss the timing of the return to work with your primary care physician, medical consultant and/or rehabilitation professional before making any decisions about returning to work. When you are ready, your GP can complete a new statement of your fitness to work indicating that you are now fit for work, taking into account the advice provided (for example, recommendations about a phased return to work, altered hours of work, amended duties, and/or workplace adaptations).

In discussion with you and with your consent, your rehabilitation professional (for example, Allied Health Professional (AHP), such as an occupational therapist or physiotherapist) can also write a clinical or AHP Health and Work Report outlining your progress and needs and recommendations for your phased return to work. This could accompany your doctor's fit note, or you can give it directly to your employer.

Before you go back to work, your employers may refer you for an occupational health assessment. This will be carried out by an occupational physician or occupational healthcare professional. They will discuss your symptoms, ask you about your job and make recommendations about readiness to return to work and recommendations to your employer about adjustments to your role.

A return-to-work meeting

It is usual for employers to arrange a return-to-work meeting. If this does not happen, you can ask for one to be set up.

Various people can be involved in such a meeting. It is likely to be with your line manager, and sometimes a representative from human resources might be present. You may also be able to request that a union representative be present, or a colleague. Depending on your company's policies, you may be able to request that a family member or your rehabilitation professional accompany you, if you feel this would be helpful.

A return-to-work plan needs to be individual to you – taking into consideration your symptoms and the impact they are having on you and your life.

Discussions in the meeting will likely cover some or all of the following:

- Your job role and how your current difficulties might affect your ability to carry out the day-to-day demands of your role.
- Discussion about your needs in the workplace, what would help and what would not.
- What adjustments can be put in place to support your to return to work.
- What gradual phasing in of hours will be put in place and what duties you could do over a set number of weeks. You may well find that the timescale needs to extend beyond what your specific employer's policy (this varies across organisations) usually allows and solutions to this need to be explored.
- How your progress will be monitored and reviewed when you are back at work.

Noting down your thoughts before the meeting about what a return-to-work plan needs to cover is often helpful.

TIPS FOR YOUR RETURN-TO-WORK MEETING
- A lot of information can be discussed in these meetings, and it can be hard to remember everything. You can ask for a summary of what was discussed, particularly if a return-to-work plan has been agreed.
- It is important to discuss the need for flexibility to be built in to your return-to-work plan. Small steps with periods of consolidation before moving on to the next step is recommended.

What are reasonable adjustments?

You and your employer need to consider together what adjustments have been advised, what might support your return to work and how these could be implemented. Some of these adjustments may be just temporary, others may need to be longer term with regular reviews. This could include:

- changing your start and finish times to avoid unnecessary energy consumption in commuting in rush hour or to fit with daily fluctuations in your energy levels;
- spacing breaks across the day and away from the workplace (e.g. sitting in your car or a local park);
- having a quiet space away from noise and interruptions in which to rest (e.g. over lunch);
- altering hours (e.g. shorter days, working part-time with days off between workdays);
- reducing workload (e.g. fewer tasks and/or more time for usual tasks);
- temporary changes to your job role or duties;
- working alongside colleagues on some tasks;
- having time off for healthcare appointments;
- adopting flexible working arrangement (e.g. working from home initially or part-time with a gradual or partial return to the office);
- provision of equipment that would help you, such as an ergonomic chair or assistive technology;
- provision of a parking space close to the building;

- strategies to manage specific difficulties (e.g. memory aids, noise-cancelling headphones);
- additional training;
- additional support (e.g. colleagues, a mentor);
- 'Access to Work' support (see box below).

ACCESS TO WORK

Access to Work is a government-run programme that provides practical advice and financial support to help overcome barriers to work for people with health conditions. The programme is flexible to try to meet the needs of the person and their job. This can include:

- physical changes to the workplace;
- specialist aids, equipment, computer software and assistive technology;
- adaptations to existing equipment;
- travel to work or while at work.

As part of your return-to-work plan, you and your employer can request an Access to Work assessment.

It is important for there to be a record of the return-to-work meetings and agreed plans. Employers vary in the level of detail of their reports of meetings, and you may be waiting for this for some time. It is therefore useful to make your own notes as soon as possible after the meeting. This will also help you to query anything that you are unsure of later. A possible format for a detailed personal record of a return-to-work plan is provided in appendix 2 for you to use as you wish.

STEP 3: Staying in work

Once you are back at work it can be easy to fall into bad habits, particularly if your return to work appears to be going well. This may include not using the strategies you originally put in place, not taking breaks, skipping lunch or eating lunch on the go, taking on too much, staying late to finish things and/or taking work home that you have been unable to complete within your hours.

You may be aware of a recurrence of some symptoms but not attribute these to changes in how you are working. Family, friends and/or work colleagues might notice that you are beginning to struggle before you become aware of this yourself. Try to remain open to their feedback.

You may need support from others (for example, work colleagues, manager or mentor) in setting and sticking to agreed boundaries in terms of both your workload and your hours of work. It is generally easier to say 'no' to taking on more work if this strays from an agreed job plan.

> **TOP TIP**
>
> Once you are back at work, you may find it helpful to write your own personal support plan to ensure that you will look after yourself and maintain progress. If you think it would be valuable for you, an example is provided below but you will need to tailor this to your individual situation.

Personal support plan

Everyday things that help me	• Pacing myself • Breaking tasks down into smaller chunks • Prioritising tasks • Using strategies I know work – e.g. to-do lists • Looking after myself – always have lunch breaks, keep hydrated
What are the things that knock me off my stride/get in the way of doing well at work? What things do I need to be aware of?	• I get engrossed and don't take breaks • I don't like saying no • I don't ask for help • Planning to do too much in my time • I forget to eat/keep hydrated
I don't seem to be managing well at work. What has changed?	• Have I stopped using my strategies? • Am I working longer hours to get through the day? • I am fatigued – am I taking regular breaks? • Has there been a change in what is expected of me or an introduction of new processes? • Have I had a change in manager or close colleague? • Has my place of work changed? • Am I feeling low, worried, or anxious? • Have things changed outside of work?

What can I do?	• Take the intiative
	• Think about what has helped in the past and restart doing it
	• Talk to my manager about what I'm finding difficult – do this early before it becomes a bigger problem
	• See my GP to talk through health concerns or to review medication
	• I'm using my strategies, but I am still struggling at work – who can I contact?

SUMMARY

- Returning to work is a key goal for most people after serious injury or illness, including Covid-19, but this can be a challenging process.

- It is important not to rush ahead with this too soon or unprepared. A planned step-by-step approach, drawing on available information and support and tailored to your individual needs, is recommended.

- This typically involves ongoing discussions about return to your job, both with your GP and any other health professionals involved and with your employer.

- There may be delays and setbacks along the way but many of these can be overcome with time and support, enabling a successful return to your previous or an amended job when you are ready to do so.

Here are two personal accounts of the challenge of return to work with Long Covid.

'I caught Covid-19 in March 2020, although I didn't know it at the time. I got steadily more unwell and after a month, I was admitted to hospital and treated for multiple micro pulmonary emboli, which had been making it hard to breathe. With medication, the most severe symptoms quickly improved, but I continued to have problems with my heart rate, recurrent fevers, chest pain and breathlessness, leading to two readmissions to hospital. Over time, things did improve, and when the new academic year started, I returned to work.

'I work in a university, teaching and writing. Before I was ill, I enjoyed running, yoga and playing with my two young children in the park. I had a full-time job that I loved. As the weeks and months went on, it was incredibly frustrating to feel that I was not recovering and indeed, that I was actually getting worse. I couldn't do the things with my children that they wanted me to, or concentrate properly on my writing. I had a sense of tiredness, of weight, that was like nothing I'd ever experienced before. Sometimes I would shake so much that I couldn't walk to my office, or even collect the children from school. Thinking, preparing lectures and teaching classes took such effort that I had to go to bed afterwards. There were periods when I felt better, and I would try to go for a run or cycle. Before Covid, these things had improved my energy and concentration. Even if it felt good to be out at the time, however, any physical exercise I tried would later make me feel exhausted and dizzy. There were days, and probably even weeks during the second national lockdown, when the combination of working and having my children at home left me so weak that I couldn't leave the house. It is very difficult to describe chronic fatigue and Long Covid. The best I can do is to say that it felt like I was being buried alive.

'I was, however, very lucky to have a doctor who referred me to a post-Covid clinic. I had one-to-one sessions with a specialist occupational therapist in chronic fatigue. First, she advised me to reduce all my activities to establish, and then maintain, a baseline where the symptoms were manageable. My doctor signed me off work, and for the first time in over a year, I stopped trying to "push through" the tiredness. Second, the occupational therapist talked me through the "pacing" and everything else that is in chapter 2 of this book. I broke my day into chunks of activities, reading, playing with the children etc. and then rested in between. I took up meditation (there's an app for that!), did breathing exercises and stretches. I worked out a daily routine and, children's lives permitting, I stuck to it. After a month, I started to feel better. After six weeks I could walk further, do more with the children, and write for short periods of time.

'I had already discussed reducing my workload with my department, but the specialist occupational therapist advised returning to work with adjustments and wrote an Allied Health Professionals Health and Work

Report outlining her recommendations. I am now increasing both my work and physical activity, very slowly, on a week-by-week basis.

'I found, and still find, managing my activity and pacing myself incredibly difficult. I do everything that is second on the list of the example of a personal support plan (I get engrossed in my work, I forget to take breaks or drink water, I hate asking for help, I hate admitting weakness and I can't say "no" to things. I always think I can do more in a day than I can). I also think that having young children creates a separate set of issues – children, in general, cannot be "paced". Overall, however, the strategies set out here have, and do, work. I know, though, that I am also very lucky. I have a loving partner and friends I can talk to. I have a job that I can do flexibly and a very supportive employer. These things enable me to (mostly) follow the advice set out in this book. As a result, I am getting stronger. My health is improving and I am regaining my sense of self. I can start to think of Long Covid as something that I am recovering from, that I will recover from. I hope that you will start to feel the same.'

In a second personal account of 'On the way back to work', it was again not until an appointment with an occupational therapist at a local Long Covid clinic after more than six months that the person began to understand and process what had happened to them:

'On the frontline of Covid there was medical and emergency triage but not much of a real sense of what was going on with those of us in the very slow lane of recovery. We had no real idea how, when or whether we would ever fully recover. Of course, people with chronic illness live with this all the time: but arriving at these questions via Covid was disorientating.

'Consults with my primary care physician and emergency doctors were able to advise on the symptoms, but they were less able to help with the things that had been lost along the way: the identity you have at work; the financial security it brings; the team you're used to working with; the things you make in your job; your bewilderment at your total lack of energy. As a long-term freelancer, I was used to living on my wits, being resourceful at times of uncertainty, but I was not prepared for the effect this illness would have on my mental health.

'Advice from the amazing occupational therapist at the Long Covid clinic around **Prioritising – Planning – Pacing** or managing my energy was when things began to turn around. Hearing that you are not alone and there were loads of others out there facing the same thing was really important, but learning about energy levels, the effort required to think, to move, to have a conversation, was stuff I'd just not had to think about before.

'Finding a baseline of things I could do was a game changer. A walk around the field every day; aiming to do just one big chore between getting up and going to bed; ordering stuff online; not sleeping all day; watching the birds on the bird feeder were some of the changes that I made.

'The early months were grim but slowly things did get better and after a few months and a little off a year after I'd first been ill, I began to ask myself the question: Can I do my job now? At one level I knew the answer was "No!" but I'd been taught ways to eke out my lower energy levels; to use my "battery" well and not let it go flat. To look after it in a way I never had. Establishing that baseline and keeping to it was the only real way to make and measure progress. Sometimes (often) I'd go too far and would go backwards – "boom and bust" in the jargon. I'd experienced this frequently on my own before help from the clinic arrived, but I now understood it and had something to work on. I had begun to know what was possible.

Through daily charts to map my energy, I developed a clear sense of where it was going and how I had to ration it for the things I really wanted to spend it on. The idea that I could make things happen or give myself energy by force of will no longer worked, even while all the time I'd hope somehow it would come and save me. I'm not saying I always managed my energy successfully but when I did do it, and kept doing it – this was what gave me my health back.

One massive advantage was working from home during the pandemic. I could work just as easily from home and in fact get so much more done; commuting would have been a lot of wasted energy when it was still in limited supply.

A second advantage was being able to work part-time on a specific project, although of course at a cost of reduced pay when *having not properly worked for more than a year I really needed to earn some money.*

'These were both decisive elements in being able to "deliver" my current work project. And as part of this, I had given myself the space and permission to have a short nap in the afternoon; go to medical appointments and work sometimes in the evenings if I'd not felt very good during the day. And no one had to know if I feel asleep in front of the TV (except my energy chart!).

'Was it easy going back to work? "No!" Were there days I wanted just to go back to bed? "Yes!" Were there times when there was more brain fog than clear thinking? "Of course!" And there were times I was sidelined as the "part-time" person when I was used to being in all the important meetings. It was part of the price that I chose to pay to make the journey back to work.

'After the project was delivered, I was beyond tired. Was my battery flat? "Yes." Did I need a rest before I could think about another project? "Yes." Do I still have to keep looking at my energy and choosing how to spend it? "Yes!" But there it was: the first post-Covid piece of work. The first money in the bank. The proof that I could still do it.'

Reviewing your job prior to return to work

The following questions are to help you talk through your work concerns. The questions are designed so that you can start thinking about your job in a focused way for yourself and in discussion with health professionals and your employer.

What are the key parts of my job?
What is my usual work pattern (e.g. hours, days, shifts etc)?
How will I get to and from work when I go back to work?
What are the demands of my job? a) Physical demands – e.g. standing, walking, climbing stairs, lifting, using tools/machinery, typing, writing, working outdoors, driving etc.   b) Thinking demands – e.g. concentrating, information overload, organising, managing, remembering etc.   c) Communication demands – e.g. using the phone, face-to-face or video conversations/meetings, report writing, giving presentations.

What symptoms do I think may cause me problems at work?

Are there any parts of the job that I think will be particularly difficult after Covid-19, or that worry me?

Are there parts of my job that I am confident I can manage?

Do I have any commitments outside of work – e.g. childcare, caring roles or study – that either affect work, or may be affected by returning to work after Covid-19?

What supervision and support did I receive in my job prior to Covid-19?

Is there anything else that is relevant to my return to work after Covid-19?

Return to work plan

Here is a possible format for a detailed personal record of a return-to-work plan.

Your name……….......................................…..….

Date of return-to-work meeting:
Present at meeting:
Job role:
Likely impact of symptoms on work:
Proposed start date for return to work:
Proposed initial pattern of working – hours/days:
Place of work:

Proposed initial workload/targets:

Proposed adjustment to support return to work:

Any other comments:

Plan agreed with:

Date progress to be reviewed:

Progress to be reviewed by:

Point of contact for support during phased return to work:

APPENDIX 3

Investigations

Not everyone we see in the Long Covid clinic needs further tests or investigations. However, sometimes they can be useful for confirming the diagnosis and checking there are no other reasons for your symptoms. Investigations may be reassuring if they are normal, but can increase anxiety if no cause for symptoms is identified. Therefore, in-depth investigations that are essentially 'tests of exclusion' (when it is considered clinically unlikely that there will be an abnormality present) should be undertaken cautiously. Nevertheless, it's often useful to run some simple screening tests (for example, blood tests to look for other causes of fatigue) with other more tailored investigations considered on a case-by-case basis.

WORD OF CAUTION

It is important to note that although tests may come back as normal, it doesn't mean that there are not biological explanations for symptoms. A normal result may be because the investigation was designed to pick up a different problem or isn't sensitive enough for Long Covid. Similarly, if an abnormality is found on a test (such as on an X-ray, computed tomography (CT) or magnetic resonance imaging (MRI) scan), it does not necessarily give us the explanation for your symptoms and may just be a coincidental finding. So, although investigations can be helpful, they need to be interpreted with care.

Many people are not sure why they are having investigations or what the results mean. What follows is a selection of the more common investigations that are sometimes considered, along with an explanation as to why they are done and what we are looking for. Please note that this is not a comprehensive list as, given the complex nature of the condition, it is beyond the scope of this book to mention them all.

Screening tests considered in Long Covid

Full blood count (FBC)

The FBC measures the blood cells circulating around the body. It looks at three types of cells, specifically red blood cells (confusingly measured by the 'haemoglobin'), white blood cells and platelets.

Haemoglobin (or Hb) – although this is a protein within red cells that binds oxygen, the Hb is used in laboratory readouts as a measure of the number of red blood cells in the body. Anaemia is the term used to describe a reduction in the number of red cells. As these cells carry oxygen to cells around your body, a fall in the quantity can contribute to or be the sole cause of fatigue. When severe (or if there has been a quick fall in the haemoglobin level), anaemia can also cause breathlessness. If anaemia is present, we would then want to look for the cause by doing further tests, which are often guided by the clinical history.

White cell count – this provides information about the immune cells circulating in the blood and the different types of cells present are quantified. In everyday clinical use, the cells of interest are the neutrophils, lymphocytes and eosinophils. As a simple guide, neutrophils target bacterial infections and are usually raised in this setting (although can also be raised in response to stress and trauma), lymphocytes provide more targeted immune responses and have immunological 'memory' in response to prior infections and vaccination (although blood lymphocyte levels are not an indicator of this), and eosinophils may be elevated in a range of conditions, including asthma and eczema (although normal values do not mean asthma is not present).

Liver and kidney function

Significant abnormalities in the functioning of the liver or kidneys can contribute to fatigue and make people feel generally unwell. Blood tests looking at the function of the kidneys and liver are therefore useful screening tests. Mild abnormalities in the results are unlikely to be the cause of symptoms, however, and may simply need to be monitored with repeat tests at an appropriate time interval. Significant or severe abnormalities that are unexpected may require specialist medical input and investigation.

Thyroid function tests

Hypothyroidism is when the thyroid gland does not produce enough thyroxine. Thyroxine is a hormone and a deficiency can cause a range of non-specific symptoms including tiredness, muscle aches, weight gain, depression and cognitive problems. So, it is important to exclude this in those with suspected Long Covid as it is easily treatable. Thyroid function tests refer to the measurement of hormones that stimulate or are produced by the thyroid gland (Thyroid stimulating hormone or TSH, and thyroxine or 'free T4').

Vitamin D

Vitamin D regulates the uptake of calcium and phosphate into the body and is important for bones, muscles and teeth. It also plays a role in maintaining a healthy immune system. Studies have suggested that vitamin D supplementation for people with ME/CFS who have low levels can improve fatigue.

Blood or urine glucose

Diabetes is a condition where the blood sugar (or glucose) levels become high due to a deficiency or abnormality in the production of the hormone insulin. Insulin enables cells in the body to take up glucose in the blood and use it for energy. People with poorly controlled diabetes can feel fatigued, washed out and non-specifically unwell. Additionally, they may become excessively thirsty and need to pass urine more frequently. Screening for diabetes involves measuring glucose in the blood or urine and is often undertaken by your primary healthcare provider.

Inflammatory markers

This includes the CRP (C-reactive protein), which is a protein produced by the liver and a marker of inflammation within the body. Infection is a cause of inflammation and the CRP is typically high in patients admitted to hospital with Covid-19 infection. Non-infective causes of an elevated CRP include chronic inflammatory conditions such as arthritis and inflammatory bowel disease. The CRP can be used to track disease activity and response to treatment, with values falling as inflammation improves. Similarly, as patients recover from Covid, the CRP typically falls. Due to the multisystem nature of Long Covid, and symptoms that overlap with recognised inflammatory diseases, the CRP can be a useful screening blood test. In our experience, however, it is usually in the normal range.

Other, more specialised blood tests should only be performed on a case-by-case basis.

Breathlessness

Investigations for breathlessness that may be considered include:

- a chest X-ray;
- a scan of the chest (a CT scan);
- lung function tests or spirometry.

Chest X-ray

A chest X-ray is often done as a screening test in people who are breathless to look for obvious abnormalities. Patients who have had Covid-19

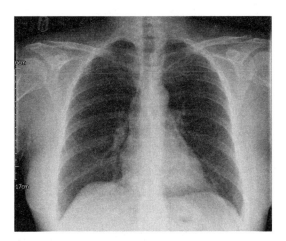

This is a chest X-ray that is completely normal and what we most commonly find in people with Long Covid who were not hospitalised. Chest X-rays are often undertaken as a screening test to look for causes of breathlessness. The X-ray also provides basic information about the heart (such as its size).

pneumonia may have persisting changes on their chest X-ray stemming from the acute infection. These lung abnormalities are not uncommon, particularly in those who had severe pneumonia, and they represent the 'footprint' of the acute infection. They typically fade over time but if persistent abnormality or 'shadowing' is seen after an interval of 12 weeks, a CT scan may be requested to look for scarring of the lung (fibrosis). If this is the case, you may be seen in a clinic specialising in lung conditions (or a dedicated post-Covid clinic). In our experience, chest X-rays in Long Covid sufferers not admitted to hospital are usually normal.

Computed tomography (CT)

A CT scan provides detailed cross-sectional images of the body (see picture below) and allows your doctor to look more closely at the structure of the lungs and other organs. It can identify whether the appearance of the lungs (and other structures within the chest) are normal or abnormal and can assess for blood clots within the blood vessels supplying the lungs (pulmonary emboli) and scarring (fibrosis) or other abnormalities of the lungs that may occur after Covid-19 pneumonia and contribute to breathlessness. The images are reviewed by a doctor specialised in imaging techniques (a radiologist).

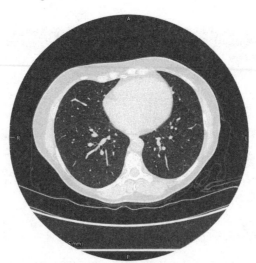

Normal CT appearance of the lungs. Chest CT scans are sometimes performed when we want a more detailed look at the lungs and the blood vessels supplying them. The scan above is a cross-section through the chest.

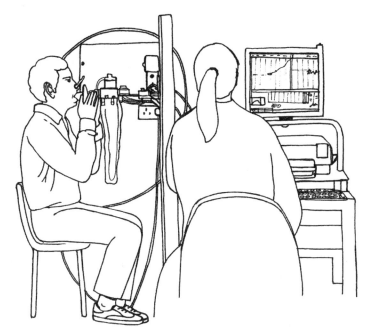

This is a diagram of a person undertaking spirometry. This procedure involves taking in the deepest breath possible, then breathing out through a tube so that we can record the volume of air you breathe out as well as the speed at which your lungs empty. You may be asked to do this a few times so we can be sure we are getting accurate measurements.

Lung function tests

To understand how well the lungs are working, as well as to look at the impact a disease is having on them, you might be asked to have spirometry or lung (pulmonary) function tests. Spirometry is a test that enables us to measure the volume of air in your lungs and how quickly the lungs can empty of air. Lung function tests include this measurement, but also measures other things, most importantly the gas transfer. This is explained in detail in the following pages.

- Spirometry – measures the volume and flow of air
- Lung function tests – measure the volume and flow of air (spirometry) and the gas transfer

Lung function tests can determine whether there is a problem with the passage of oxygen through the airways, into the airspaces and across the lining of the lung into the surrounding blood vessels. Different components of the breathing tests can provide information about the nature and location of the abnormality (if detected). This is particularly important if your doctor suspects you may have scarring of the lungs (fibrosis), which may hamper the uptake of oxygen into your body.

In our experience, despite persistent breathlessness, lung function assessments are usually within the 'normal range' for individuals not hospitalised with Covid-19. Normal range refers to values that fall within the accepted limits of normality for individuals of the same gender, age, height and ethnicity.

Occasionally, these breathing tests can identify people with asthma or other airway or lung conditions (either as cause for symptoms or contributing to symptoms), which will allow your doctor to start appropriate treatment for this, alongside management of your Long Covid. Abnormalities in the lung function results may also highlight the need for further investigations – this is beyond the scope of this book.

You might see lung function tests quoted in clinic letters to your primary healthcare provider and note that there is rarely a clear explanation as to why the tests were arranged and what the results actually mean. The following text breaks down the components of the test to explain what each part means and what we're looking for. Don't worry if you don't understand it – this is here just for interest/background information.

FVC

FVC stands for 'forced vital capacity' and is a measure of the total volume of air that you can breathe out after taking in the deepest breath that you can. This gives us an idea of the size (or rather volume) of your lungs. Some conditions, such as those affecting the lungs themselves (a group of diseases known as interstitial lung diseases), can reduce the ability of the lungs to expand normally and therefore the amount of air that is breathed out is lower than expected for someone of the same age and gender with healthy lungs.

Occasionally, Covid-19 pneumonia can result in persisting lung abnormalities and this test can provide information on how the lungs have

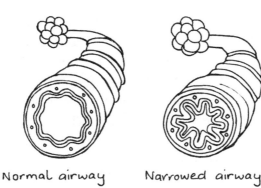

Normal airway   Narrowed airway

Conditions affecting the airways, such as asthma or viral-induced inflammation, can result in the airways becoming narrowed, which may make breathing difficult. When we assess this using spirometry, we look at the FEV1, which gives us an idea about the speed of air emptying through the airways, and how this compares to the lung volume overall (FVC). A FEV1/FVC ratio of less than 0.7 suggests airways narrowing (referred to as 'obstruction').

been affected. In most people, the FVC improves in line with their clinical recovery, but in a small proportion who have persisting lung scarring/fibrosis, the value may remain reduced. In these instances, people may be followed up and monitored in a respiratory clinic.

FEV1

FEV1 stands for 'forced expiratory volume in 1 second' and refers to the amount of air that is breathed out of your lungs in the first second after you have taken a deep breath in and breathed out hard and fast. It gives an idea of how quickly the lungs can empty of air, and the speed at which air moves from the air sacs (alveoli) along the airways (air tubes) and out of the body. This speed depends on the airway's calibre or size. If the airways are narrowed, such as in asthma or COPD (chronic obstructive pulmonary disease), then less air empties out in the first second and the value of the FEV1 is lower than what would be expected for someone of the same age and gender with normal airways.

FEV1/FVC ratio

The FEV1/FVC ratio is sometimes quoted in medical reports or clinical correspondence you might be sent. As the FEV1 gives us an idea about the speed of air emptying out from the lungs (the airflow) and the FVC provides a measure of lung volume, the ratio can help us see if there is a problem with the airways – that is, whether they are narrowed or 'obstructed', causing air to travel more slowly out of the lungs. If the ratio is lower than normal, we call this 'airways obstruction'. This is important in assessing patients with suspected COPD or asthma (both conditions affecting the airways). Inflammation and hyper-reactivity of the airways ('over-sensitive' airways) can also be an after-effect of respiratory viral infections, including Covid-19, and may present in a similar way to asthma.

If the ratio is high, then air is emptying out of the lungs quickly. This may be normal but can indicate a different type of problem, referred to as a 'restrictive pattern'. This is seen in diseases affecting the lung tissue (including lung fibrosis), as well as conditions where there is a problem with fully expanding the chest wall (such as when the muscles around the chest are weak).

In individuals who did not require hospital admission during their acute Covid infection, the FEV1, FVC and the FEV1/FVC ratio are usually within normal range.

The gas transfer (quoted as TLCO/DLCO)

- TLCO stands for the transfer factor of the lung for carbon monoxide.
- DLCO stands for the diffusion capacity of the lung for carbon monoxide.

(They are the same thing.)

The gas transfer (TLCO/DLCO) provides a measure of how well gas can cross the lining of the lung (more specifically, the air sacs or alveoli) into the surrounding blood vessels. The test involves you breathing in a small amount of carbon monoxide and then holding your breath. The gas travels through the airways, into the lung tissue, and is absorbed into your blood. When breathing back out, any remaining carbon monoxide within the lung is measured. We use carbon monoxide (CO) for this test because it is easier to measure than oxygen, and when CO transfer is reduced, it is likely that oxygen transfer is also reduced.

Conditions that affect the lining of the lung (such as lung fibrosis, where there is thickening of the air sacs) or the blood vessels within the lung (such as pulmonary emboli) reduce the ability of the gas to be absorbed and therefore more carbon monoxide is breathed out. This is then converted into a numerical value alongside a percentage and compared to a predicted 'normal' value for age and gender. A range of between 80 and 120 per cent is considered normal. This test can show some variability from one day to the next and subtle changes in values need to be interpreted with care.

Other investigations

Occasionally, investigations looking at the heart are arranged. This may be to investigate the feeling of the heart racing (or palpitations), breathlessness, chest pains or symptoms that raise a concern regarding a heart problem unrelated to Covid.

Electrocardiogram (ECG)

An ECG is a common test that records the electrical activity of your heart. It allows measurement of the heart rate (how fast your heart is going) and rhythm (whether it is pumping regularly or irregularly).

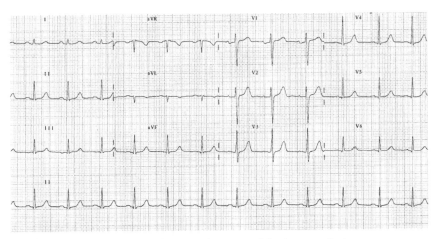

This trace is a recording of the electrical activity of the heart, called an electrocardiogram or ECG. In people with Long Covid, the ECG is typically normal.

Holter monitoring

A Holter monitor is a type of portable electrocardiogram (ECG), which records the electrical activity of your heart continuously over 24 hours or longer. Cardiac electrodes (small patches that stick to the skin) are placed on your chest and are connected to a small monitoring box by wires. You will go home with this monitor in place and the heart's rate and rhythm will be recorded while you perform your normal daily activities. The reading is then downloaded and interpreted by the cardiology team, who will feed back the result to your doctor.

Echocardiogram (echo)

An echocardiogram is an ultrasound scan assessment of your heart and gives a measure of the heart's pumping ability (your cardiac function), the pressures on the different sides of the heart and the connections between the chambers of the heart (the valves). When the heart is not pumping as efficiently as it could, this is referred to as 'heart failure' and may result in symptoms such as breathlessness during activity and fatigue. Reassuringly, though, people with Long Covid who were not hospitalised have not been found to be at any more risk of heart abnormalities than the general population.

REFERENCES AND RESOURCES

Chapter 1

National Institute for Health Research (2021) 'Living with Covid-19 – second review'. https://evidence.nihr.ac.uk/themedreview/living-with-covid19-second-review/

Khamsi, R. (2021) 'Rogue antibodies could be driving severe Covid-19'. *Nature*. https://www.nature.com/articles/d41586-021-00149-1

UKRI (2021) 'The immune system and Long Covid'. https://www.ukri.org/our-work/tackling-the-impact-of-covid-19/understanding-coronavirus-covid-19-and-epidemics/the-immune-system-and-long-covid/

NIH (2021) 'Coronavirus and the nervous system'. https://www.ninds.nih.gov/Current-Research/Coronavirus-and-NINDS/nervous-system#nervoussystem

Iacobucci, G. (2020) 'Long Covid: Damage to multiple organs presents in young, low risk patients'. *BMJ*, 371. https://doi.org/10.1136/bmj.m4470

Pretorius, E., Vlok, M., Venter, C. et al (2021) 'Persistent clotting protein pathology in Long COVID/Post-Acute Sequelae of COVID-19 (PASC) is accompanied by increased levels of antiplasmin'. *Cardiovasc Diabetol* 20, 172. https://doi.org/10.1186/s12933-021-01359-7

Chapter 2

Royal College of Occupational Therapists, 'How to conserve your energy: Practical advice for people during and after having Covid-19' (www.rcot.co.uk/files/conserving-your-energy-practical-advice-people-during-and-after-having-covid-19pdf).

Pemberton S. and Berry, C. (2009) *Fighting Fatigue* (London: Hammersmith Press).

Chapter 3

Clifton-Smith, T. (2021) *How To Take A Breath* (Auckland, NZ: Random House.)

Physiotherapy for breathing pattern disorders resources for physiotherapists (physiotherapyforbpd.org.uk).

Breathing Pattern Disorders Hyperventilation Syndromes (bradcliff.com).

British Lung Foundation: Coronavirus and Covid-19 (blf.org.uk).

Chapter 4

www.sleepio.com/ (general sleep resource).

www.blf.org.uk/support-for-you/osa (information on OSA).

sleep-apnoea-trust.org/ (Information on OSA).

For further information on OSA see www.blf.org.uk/support-for-you/osa or the Sleep Apnoea Trust Association website https://sleep-apnoea-trust.org/

Chapter 5

Moving Medicine https://movingmedicine.ac.uk/

Chapter 6

Naidu, S.B, Shah, A.J, Saigal, A., Smith, C., Brill, S.E., Goldring, J., Hurst, J.R., Jarvis, H., Lipman, M., Mandal, S. (2021) 'The high mental health burden of "Long Covid" and its association with on-going physical and respiratory symptoms in all adults discharged from hospital', *European Respiratory Journal*, DOI: 10.1183/13993003.04364-2020

Daher, A., Cornelissen, C., Hartmann, N.-U., Balfanz, P., Müller, A., Bergs, I., Aetou, M., Marx, N., Marx, G., Simon, T.-P., Müller-Wieland, D., Hartmann, B., Kersten, A., Müller, T., Dreher, M. (2021) 'Six months follow-up of patients with invasive mechanical ventilation due to Covid-19 related ARDS', *International Journal of Environmental Research and Public Health*, 18, DOI: 10.3390/ijerph18115861

Finding a therapist:
In the UK, appropriately qualified therapists should be registered with the Health and Care Professions Council (www.hcpc-uk.org). You can find a psychologist via the British Psychological Society (www.bps.org.uk) and Cognitive Behaviour Therapists via the British Association for Behavioural and Cognitive Psychotherapy (babcp.com). Counsellors can be found via the British Association for Counselling and Psychotherapy (www.bacp.co.uk).

Relaxation links:
Mindfulness:
Find a mindfulness therapist: www.accessmbct.com
Mindfulness teachers and events: www.mindfuldirectory.org

Single relaxation techniques:
Progressive muscle relaxation – numerous resources online from various NHS trusts.
Deep/abdominal or diaphragmatic breathing – numerous resources online from various NHS trusts and others (see www.nhs.uk for basic advice).
Imagery/visualisation – numerous resources online. Many prefer guided visualisation that can be accessed via popular apps such as HeadSpace.

Chapter 8

Popkirov, S., Staab, J.P., Stone, J. (2017) 'Persistent postural-perceptual dizziness (PPPD): a common, characteristic and treatable cause of chronic dizziness', BMJ, 18(1). http://dx.doi.org/10.1136/practneurol-2017-001809

Chapter 9

www.som.org.uk/covid-19-return-work-guide-recovering-workers
www.som.org.uk/covid-19-return-work-guide-managers
www.yourcovidrecovery.nhs.uk/your-road-to-recovery/returning-to-work/
www.gov.uk/government/publications/the-fit-note-a-guide-for-patients-and-employees/the-fit-note-guidance-for-patients-and-employees
www.gov.uk/access-to-work
www.equalityhumanrights.com
acas.org.uk
www.disabilityrightsuk.org
www.gov.uk/browse/benefits
www.citizensadvice.org.uk/
benefitsandwork.co.uk

ABOUT THE CONTRIBUTORS

Dr Emily Fraser is a Consultant in Respiratory Medicine at Oxford University NHS Foundation Trust. Her clinical and research background is in Interstitial Lung Disease and she is the clinical lead for the Post-Covid Assessment Clinic. Since its formation in July 2020, the service has grown to incorporate multiple specialists to enable the holistic assessment and management of patients with post-Covid complications. She is committed to advancing medical understanding of Long Covid and is working on both national and local research projects to investigate potential mechanisms driving symptoms following Covid.

Dr Anton Pick is a consultant in Rehabilitation Medicine and Clinical Lead at the Oxford Centre for Enablement, a regional specialist rehabilitation centre and part of Oxford University Hospitals NHS Foundation Trust. Anton is the Clinical Lead for Long Covid for NHS England in the South East of England. He has a special interest in managing complex disability and rehabilitation, and aiding recovery. He is committed to raising the standard of care for Long Covid sufferers through research and advocacy. Anton is a co-investigator in one of the largest Long Covid NIHR funded studies in the UK.

Rachael Rogers is a Specialist Occupational Therapist. She has an MSc in mental health and since graduating has worked in a variety of occupational therapy roles in the NHS. She is a specialist in fatigue management and regularly delivers training for doctors and other health professionals on practical strategies to manage fatigue. She is the Clinical Lead of the community chronic fatigue service in Oxfordshire, which she co-established in 2005. She is a member of the multi-disciplinary Post-Covid Assessment Clinic and rehabilitation team in Oxford, working with both patients and NHS staff affected by Long Covid.

Emma Tucker is a specialist respiratory physiotherapist and co-manager of the Community Respiratory Team in Oxford Health NHS Foundation Trust. She has a Masters in Cardiorespiratory Physiotherapy and has spent her career working with patients with acute and long-term respiratory conditions. Emma is a passionate advocate for patients with Long Covid and spearheaded the establishment of the Oxfordshire Post-Covid Rehabilitation Service and leads the Oxfordshire Post-Covid Rehabilitation Pathway.

Dr Daniel Zahl is a Consultant Clinical Psychologist and accredited CBT therapist and supervisor. After studying Experimental Psychology at Oxford, he went on to complete a doctorate in Clinical Psychology. Since qualifying in 2005 he has worked with people with chronic physical health problems in the NHS and with people with mental health problems in private practice. He provides teaching, training and supervision, and has written a number of book chapters and published in peer reviewed journals. His areas of specialist interest include chronic fatigue, bariatric surgery, diabetes and more recently Long Covid, where he is part of the Post-Covid Assessment Clinic.

Dr Suleman Latif is a specialist registrar in Sports and Exercise Medicine in Oxford. He completed the MSc Sport and Exercise Medicine at Queen Mary University of London, and has peer-reviewed publications and presentations in the areas of public health, global health, medical education and sports medicine.

Ruth Tyerman is a specialist vocational rehabilitation occupational therapist with over 30 years' experience. She was the team lead for a specialist brain injury vocational rehabilitation programme and has supported other services in developing vocational rehabilitation for people with brain injury as well as complex trauma. She continues to provide specialist training, supervision and mentoring to occupational therapists providing vocational rehabilitation after brain injury, and also now provides support to staff of the Post-Covid Assessment Clinic.

Dr Christopher Turnbull is an NIHR Clinical Lecturer in Respiratory Medicine with the University of Oxford and the Oxford University Hospitals NHS Foundation Trust. He is an expert in sleep disorders and conducts research into finding new treatments for patients with obstructive sleep apnoea. He is an investigator in a research study looking at the impact of Covid-19 on different patient groups, including those with cancer and sleep disorders. He is a co-investigator in clinical trials evaluating the role of new treatments for Covid-19.

Christine Kelly is founder of the AbScent charity and has experienced smell loss herself several times. Her initial loss in 2012 led her on a journey of recovery that lasted eight years, during which she researched anosmia and smell training and established a Facebook page to share her knowledge. Following the formation of AbScent, the community has grown exponentially as a result of the pandemic and as of 2021 stands at over 75k members worldwide. She is a Research Associate at the University of Reading and a Research Fellow at the Centre for the Study of the Senses, Institute of Philosophy, University of London.

Dr Helen Davies is a Consultant Respiratory Physician in the University Hospital of Wales. Her research background is in Pleural Disease. She is Clinical Lead for the Pleural and Post-Covid Respiratory Clinics. She is committed to improving knowledge of potential underlying mechanisms for Long Covid and the care of Long Covid sufferers. She is a Co-Investigator in several national and international Long Covid research studies.

Emily Jay is a Clinical Specialist Physiotherapist at the South London and Maudsley NHS Trust. She is a neurological physiotherapist and a committee member for the Association of Chartered Physiotherapists with an Interest in Vestibular Rehabilitation (ACPIVR). Within an out-patient setting, she supports patients suffering with dizziness and imbalance following Covid-19 infection.

Lisa Burrows is a Consultant Physiotherapist working for Mersey Care NHS Foundation Trust and work in both the local hospitals and community. She leads the ENT Balance Clinic and sees people with dizziness and balance disorders in the Southport and Ormskirk area. She is the education sub-committee chair for the Association of Chartered Physiotherapists with an Interest in Vestibular Rehabilitation (ACPIVR).

Dr Andrew Lewis is a Clinical Lecturer in Cardiovascular Medicine at the University of Oxford. In addition to consulting with adults with a range of heart conditions, he conducts research using new imaging techniques to find better ways to detect and treat inflammation and its consequences in human heart tissue.

Dr Rohan Wijesurendra is a Clinical Lecturer in Cardiovascular Medicine. He commenced Cardiology specialist training in Oxford and completed a DPhil (PhD) in 2018. His clinical and research interests are in the fields of arrhythmia and catheter ablation, cardiac magnetic resonance imaging (MRI), and clinical trials.

Dr Julia Newton is a Consultant in Rheumatology/Sport and Exercise Medicine at the Oxford University Foundation Hospitals Trust, a Senior Sports Physician for the English Institute of Sport and holds an Honorary post at the University of Oxford. She is the Head of School of Medicine for Thames Valley, Chair of the Specialty Advisory Committee for SEM and Vice-President of Faculty of Sport and Exercise Medicine. She is an advisory member of the Post-Covid multi-disciplinary team.

Dr Christopher Speers completed higher specialist training in Sport and Exercise Medicine in the West Midlands. He is a Consultant in Sport and Exercise Medicine, working at the Nuffield Orthopaedic Centre, Oxford with the Oxsport and complex Musculoskeletal teams. He is an advisory member of the Post-Covid multi-disciplinary team.

Dr Andy Tyerman is a Consultant Clinical Neuropsychologist. Since qualifying as a clinical psychologist in 1979, he worked initially in in-patient and then in community neurorehabilitation. From 1992 to 2020 he developed and led the Community Head Injury Service in Buckinghamshire. He continues to undertake research, supervise, teach and write on community and vocational rehabilitation after brain injury and is also a trustee of Headway UK and the Vocational Rehabilitation Association.

Additional contributions from

Dr Kim Rajappan (Consultant Cardiologist, Oxford University NHS Foundation trust)

Dr Annabel Nickol (Consultant in Sleep Medicine, Oxford University NHS Foundation Trust)

Dr Tylan Yukselen (Consultant in Psychological Medicine, Oxford University NHS Foundation Trust)

Dr Nick Talbot (Respiratory Consultant, Oxford University NHS Foundation Trust)

Professor Jane Parker (Founder and Director of the Flavour Centre, University of Reading)

The Oxfordshire Post-Covid Rehabilitation team: Victoria Masey, Kerrie Crowley, Catherine Clayton, Rebecca Prower, Rachel Lardner, Amanda Neophytou, Lisa Johnson, Jill Brooks, Kelly Mclaughlin

Lizzie Grillo on behalf of Physiotherapy for Breathing Pattern Disorders

Tania Clifton-Smith on behalf of the BradCliff Breathing Method™

ACKNOWLEDGEMENTS

This book would not exist without the input of the people we've seen in at the Post-Covid Assessment Clinic, Oxford and elsewhere in the UK. With particular thanks for the quotes, contributions and feedback to: Amelia Sayce; Jean Postlethwaite-Dixon; Valerie Knight; Katrina Stevens; Aoife Mannix; Toni Waknell; Deborah Orr; David Hockaday; Amy Tandy; Nell Freeman-Romilly; Linden Baxter; Lucia Mackay; Michael Osborne; Lisa Marie Mclane; Julia Woolley; Holly Atkins; Shaked Ashkenazi; Mark Turner and Catherine Briddick.

The authors would like to thank their professional colleagues, friends and families who contributed their valuable support, time and expertise to the creation of this book. In no particular order: Dr Ahmad Saif; Professor Tim Nicholson; Shelley and Michael Pick; Dr Nayia Petousi; Dr Susannah Brain; Dr Alex Novak; Professor Kyle Pattinson; Professor Fergus Gleeson; Paul Swan; Jodie Summers; Sarah Broadway; Paul Tucker; Mike Cuerden; Aparna Zahl; Julian Ball; Daniel Rogers; Sanna Nabi; Zoë Blanc and Charlotte Croft.

The '3 Ps' terminology appears in Chapter 2 by kind permission of The Royal College of Occupational Therapists. BradCliff Breathing™ practices and methods appear in Chapter 3 by kind permission of Tania Clifton-Smith. The Borg CR scale® (CR10) © Gunnar Borg, 1982, 1998, 2004) appears in Chapter 5 with permission. The scale and full instruction can be obtained through BorgPerception www.borgperception.se

INDEX